To Hear the Heart, to Hear the Sea

Paul Fearne

chipmunkapublishing
the mental health publisher

Published by
Chipmunkapublishing
United Kingdom

http://www.chipmunkapublishing.com

ISBN : 9781782827039

This book is a short novel written in poetic prose. It alternates between long stanzas and shorter stanzas; each type of stanza arrangement being divided by chapter numbers. This structure gives the book a feeling of ebb and flow and pulse, just as the sea, just as a heart.

Paul Fearne

4

Chapter 1.

And then, there was nothing left – nothing but a heart, a heart pounding. What do we say now? Say now, to it all? The signs regret nothing, and that which has movement does not stand in disarray. Do not belittle us, the time is of the making. I will not shun, for that is the way of all ways. I am one to carry, carry the lantern in the strength of all moulds. There is a time, one that doesn't ring the line. As much as we would like to, we come without full glasses. But what is this anyway, but the languishing of hope?

But wait, there is a chance, coming from behind, and through all roads. Do not bend for the wind, concentrate yourself, and what is pleasant will rise, and then fall. I have known many of the things we encounter, known their breeze and their desire. Can there be a wisdom that dries all wounds? In one sense, there is a swing that levies no faults. But what of the rest? The rest that seeps in abandon. I will find you. It will not take long.

Listen to the wind, it tells a story. Deep within, and then without. The sea is here, but what is not remiss is the fun we have in the yard. There is nothing like this, nothing that harbours fate with such fellowship. Writing on our limbs – there is something more. There is a catching, that with random aplomb, seeks more of the masonry on the way. I have listened, now where is my reward? It is in the eves, where all good things go to be.

And all the while things seemed strange. Not strange of course in the normal fashion, but that strange in the course of things that has no respite to carry, nor bidden to warrant. Do not depend on the wire that tells us our enemies are dry, or the falconry is at liberty to dive. There can be no other way than this. This is the way we must jar in the bagel. Come now, there is nothing past the repartee. And then, quiet and shrewd.

And without thought, the senses arise to take the day. 'We are not with them', I hear you say. But in the meantime, a laugh erupts – one that that does not settle easily. And in this laugh is the world, in this laugh is what is best. I think of things deeper, and know that the time it takes to wrestle a star-crust through the window of life is not what we should expect. We find ourselves awakened, to something fresh, to something new.

Do tell – tell of ramblings made a-right, and then let us see things as they really are. I am of the time, of the place, of the well, and of the spring. The forwards we have knows no reverse. And then, like a wind that does not sing for the crowd, a happiness descends – boo says the crowd, hooray says the wind. I will have only what is left, and then a larger piece of the forging of strains. Come, in this we are equals. There can only be what the sands tell of.

There was once a thistle, that grew in times of trouble. And there it lay, as if by chance. And then, in thickest groom, it went on its way – ever increasing, until! The look from its demise filtered down in unruly smocks, and damage-less pieces. But what of it now? It swims in tides of golden tangles, and knows that when the finish of the walk is seen, there will be a golden grace to soothe the embers. Do not look back, the hearth needs cleaning.

And then, like a lyre-bird running – something shifting in the sands will be found. But now, and afterwards, a sense that the hardship has been faced, and the knowing of such things will paint a picture – we will hear a distant cry, that muffles the wind seeking allurement. But what of this, when the heart knows which way to be beat, and the sea laughs out aloud? There is life still to be lived, and magic to be strode. Come now let us be adventured filled.

A systematic appraisal blooms, and like the orchid of ourselves, a running takes hold, that can neither further the bettering, nor come last in the race. Be that as it may, we see through the flesh, and bone, and symptomatic nuances. Drive further, it will not hurt. I am one to see things lurch to the fore. We cannot see things in the dark, that much is a conduit, to all things. Please be plenty, much is here to be with you.

There was once a sound, that grated on dirt. And in this sound, much was heard, and much was not. But here, where the sands of yore envision warn out particles of life, there is a chance to glean, and a chance to surmise. We will know this to be one with the life of it. I will sing a register higher for your pleasure. And can this be all – something that is not of this world? Do not play the sands, they will not wreak. Come now, a furthering will commence.

And then, light as a light from the tethers, a hand stitched bow – one that folds in on itself, and has as its ranch the milestones of an age. Do not linger, all that is left is the movement of resonance. Do not delay, what we know to be inside, is that which flounders on servitude. I am one to bring the kitchen, and all that will come to pass. Most surprising is the levity, and the fetching of scraps for the times. Do not be one to fetch the rounds, there can only be a similitude of sounds.

Without a whisper, all things come, and then stride forth, nearing completion. There is never a grain of sand left, but what of the nearest thing? The thing that harbours all. The thing that launches, as it dismisses. Be like a time piece when you can, but otherwise take kindly to things. Are we here? – Do we whisper like the rest of it? A snore here, a drawl there. And when we diminish, we love, and in that motion, a cautionary tale. We will include…

And like all vessels the sea has them. And here, we say, with salutations in hand, a joyous farewell. Do not feel sorry for us, we are here to travel. But what is left? What is far-gone? There can never be anything more. We accost the night, only because it is in range. There is a longing here, that has as its surety enough to classify. I will not linger, until whispers form words, and the heart is rendered motionless. Be that as it may – we must continue.

And now – what is left? What is left in the guts so that they ooze drive. Can there be compensation? We will never know. We must pursue, and in pursuing right a wrong. And then, something that is remiss. Can we grasp at the fibres of it, and know it to be there before the very touch of this existence? I will not stop, for all the vinegar of the world. And here where the sands do not smart, we have come for something, something else. And what else is that? We will never know.

Without a thought, some things congeal, and others reminisce. There is a space through the clouds, that pertains to no endeavour, and nothing left as a windfall. There are tokens here, that sense no fruit, and belong in and of themselves. A tutelage to the morrow, and all it stands for. I believe in one thing, and one thing only – we have a heart, and it pulses.

There is, in the here and now, a vantage through the trees – one we can never feel ourselves more alone that this. But when we fly, we do so with speed, and utmost compulsion. There is nothing else we can do. I believe in a second thing, the sea lives. But what of the sand, in roundabouts and turtle colours? There is now a testing of the waters, we should dive in, and see ourselves lightning quick, as the covers of books. What is this – we are free.

A pitch, to the left, and off we go. There are times when the sands of life diminish. But here in the returning of the harbour to the depths, we see the love we have for the sky. What is more, a heralding that traces itself on votive flooring never knows which way to turn. We cannot consider ourselves lucky, for in this there is an inch to give. And when we give it, sense reigns in shards of glass, and the two movements of the wind – back and forward - come to strengthen, and then turn.

Having a hold on so much – there is a richness in life to be savoured. And it is our solemn duty to be the ones to ring things through. I love the feeling – the feeling we get when all is made, and the night and her vespers give nonchalance as a freedom to curtail. What the sempiternal ravages of the phrase have in store for the window. We love it here, where the rain does not speak, and the silence of the vagabondage delivers a truce. Come and be a part of it.

There is a part of us that cannot see, and a part that can. And when we look, one part or the other looks out. But when we don't look, we feel our very eyes disregarded. But this is okay. For looking requires the heart, and with it, the stumbling blocks of life. Do not tempt me, the singing we do will not stop us. But now, when silence pertains to mystery, there belongs a canter to our journey, that simply revels in it. Stand close, it is all we can do.

What of the day? How do we ascertain our vision? There is here, an unnerving, one that bodes no time afresh. We see, and the curbs of prescience rely – rely on us. Do not believe in shadows, they come to harvest. But what we have now touched, is the detritus, and the goad. There is a sense that hope can win, once again. Do not right the ship, it is here for the time it takes. And that time is all. Come now, there is a way through, as there is a way up.

There is now a time for farce. There is now a time for vindication. There is now – well something. And it is this something that perplexes us, and leaves us drained. Do not temper the worrying about things, it lifts, as it unfolds. Come now, we cannot speak in this way. Because it is here, that the encumbered languish, and the desperation of an age tests itself against the rock. Do not feel the semblance, of here to there and back again. We will not stop.

And when the dawn sang anew, there was a
template there to follow. And follow it we will.
Crouching, and lounging and being solid in the
remorse of it all. I have never known such calm –
did it last? There were times, in the wind, in the
breeze. A lagoon, and factory of the still-hearted. I
am relishing the silence of it all. It is as if I had
started again, and found the recipe for the fruit
from the tree. Come now, solace will be no issue.
We must parade once more.

As soon as we lost sight of it, as soon as the trail
that blazed could not be noticed, a far-away
sound. In depth, as in night, things in contrition. I
have never known light, light from the candle stick,
light from the dimensions of things. Have you
heard the cry, the cry from the stables? It is like
nothing else. And when we know its source, we
can find ourselves pushing, pushing back the rails.
But what is more, we are here to see, to see in
new ways. We won't call time.

And, like the style of an igloo, there arose
something in the mist. What was that thing? Was it
like nothing we had seen before (or after for that
matter)? Come now, there are answers, and there
are guesses, and we have both. Do not try to steal
the layers we have. For in them are the folds of
life, and here, we seek no redress. I will not see
you until you say when – and then only when you
have written deeply, of things to come, and things
to be. Yes, things to be.

Moistening our eyes a little, we see with a depth that astounds. Remove the water, and there is left a direct line of sight to the heart. What more is left, is not what we expected. Hearts and dire conundrums. There is here imbued with life a certain intractable insistence – and this here is us – as we follow the route down through the aeons. Do not prefigure what we mean to do, it is only here we really flourish. Come and seek the corner – we will be sound.

Shine through – shine through it all. When we have had enough, we will say so. I am stirring, stirring the paint viscous. And here where we love to be, feelings that arise, that have no tenderness, but are revered through the whole in the wall. Can we see ourselves here? What do we see? A face seen with age. And here, where the lives of us all co-mingle, we shed a tear for the life we lead. What is more, we have a handle on things, despite all and sundry. Sweet all.

Have we found it yet? Have we found what we are looking for? It is here. Here within us. All we must do is look, and lo, it is found. But so simple? That much is true. And then, a longing that does not escape. We are here, here like never before. I have the igloo by my side, and here with bountiful array, the life we lead can bring us there. There are no tricks, and no party games. The only thing we need, that we can't bring with us, is luck. Share your source.

Bring all-and-sundry – and see that they are alert, and leaving no dirt. I will fashion a wig, one that has only centimetres to roam. And here, like a rooftop that does not shade, a far outcrop menaces all who come through. But what is its domain? What is its structure? There can be more to carry here than we at first believed. But do not stand for it – we must pursue ends, and not simplicities. Come for the shoreline, there is not the harbour there.

A mismatch of lives – coming through, coming down. And then a spark, and then something else, anew. I found something for them, and it says phew. A certain pleasant cart carries them to the next stop. Much laughter, and guffaws, and all that will be. Do not sense the way, use your eyes. And in this way, temples will be built, and offices will sustain us. And then, like a long field, a motion that harbours something more. We will see again.

There is much said to tide the windings over. But we are interested in something cold, and off the shoulder. And much to the Samson of it – we visit, but without much due respect, we carry our luggage back through the streets, and know our selves to be tame. What is there missing? What is there sought for, more than is angled? I have fought, for the strangeness of things to win, but in this there is that which comes with pieces. Do not be disappointed in the levering of summer fruits. When I marry the sky, I will have ochre.

There are places that have as their repute the cold glass of fibres. And then, like the solstice in winter sand, much comes from the lineament. We have never left behind anyone or anything, but now we come for the fjord, that knows of earth's rumbling, and senses the trail by the way. I have found here something that the juncture would allow. And in this movement from here to there, space, and the traction to keep going. There can be nothing more.

And then, like a trance that knows only itself, a well-spring comes, and has as the ages of it much renown. I have found a way through. I have found a way through. Have a sense of where you are going, believe in something, or somethings, be prepared for an adventure, and then simply walk into life. There is no greater movement, from here to there. And then, just relax, and feel your way forward. Everything comes.

An apogee for the sky. Thoughts that never linger. What we described as boisterous, could never be. Be the window that looks out onto so much. And then in time to a lullaby of its own choosing, we fend off diligence, and know sight to be something that would be useful. And then, like water over sand, a lost memory returns, and invigorates us, so that we feel again, and know this time to be one of great heart and greater subsistence.

What gives the scene its luminescence? What gives us the strength to enjoy the journey? And here, nestled in close, there is a wire of exacting might. A wire that trembles in the water, and does not surface for air at any point. There are surfaces, and there are surfaces. And then there is this, here, that eats the tiredness in all of us. Let us be pleasant, and then outstrip ourselves through the garden gate and beyond. There can be no commotion.

Considering the options ahead, we chose to go straight. And that we did. And then without a thought of care for ourselves, we wandered close to the pathway, and saw our sense of pride diminish. But of the thought for it, that trembles in rain. I have no other thought than this – to continue.

Chapter 2.

There is a place, in every beating heart. There is a sound in every motion of the sea. There is here, every want of every fibre of everybody that has ever swam. There is an imprint on each our foreheads as we stride forth. And that we will do.

Considering where we came from, something special has happened. And that something special is life. And that something special is around us, in all its forms. I believe in one refrain, and that is the here and now.

Wishing the charm would stay. And it has! There is never a moment too soon – too soon, too soon, to embark on the journey. And then, a masquerade without the tails, or the frills. I am never too tired for this. Come and see.

A realm, despite everything. I will wish for more, and the entry is despite. Comfortable, and all that is pleasing. There is never a time like this. We must grasp it and feel endeared by it. We have come full circle, and then what remains.

Catching on, we feel what no one has felt – no one has felt in the long stretch of it. A mission to be sure, but what is that? We come for the strangeness, and stay for the life of it. And then it is here, much to our pleasure.

Feeling languid, or not feeling at all. This is in the fallout from nothingness. And where are we now? We have come to that state of non-regress, that features the hills and the sand. Do not despise here, things are at their premium.

A listening the trees do, to cast a shadow in the beyond. And here, where along-side of us there is wonder – wandering wonder – there is the moon that has no side, and no place to be. We have seen the stars, now let us see what else.

And afterward, there was the noise of soldiers. From where it came, nobody could tell. And then a brisky walk, and all that is left, we will never know. Could the legions be the things that save us; in the end?

Moisture – rising. Simplicity, moving. There are times in amongst it, times when we cannot run. And then, like a gulp of air, magic. Magic through everything we hold dear. And then, like a wind that never ceases -a new sense of what it is right.

Formidable, and alive – formidable and attuned. We race for what is next – that is the way of it. Never be the crowd, it only calls. Never be what is in-between – maybe for a while. There will be more to say, and we will say it.

And then there was more to savour. And within, and without – keeping pace, and walking slowly. We navigate the impasse with strength and courage. And then, like a turbulence through thin air, we sail again – yes, again.

Bestowing a sense of right into things. And then, like a radish in the parlour, we do not know where to sit. But what we have found, will amuse us all. There are times that are through, and times that know no commiseration. This much is true.

Lessening the blow, the blow of all things. What catches is nice to have known. What fallows, is a tempest in rear-guard. We solemnly remember all that has been, and all that has become. Do not differentiate, there are silhouettes to be had.

Cascading through, and in-between. Through, and in-between. There is nothing left like it. And here, where the swans of forever talk of majesty, more musings than a rival could bear. What is this now? We will see.

Missing a beat, but coming through. All the fabrics are tethered, this much we can see. And then, like a fire in the woods, a cascading that never remits. Do not be the one to settle – to settle is to score. Make much of it, I implore.

Caustic, and without recourse. Never settle, only if we must. And here, where the silence triggers something deeper, we lunge forward, and know our bones to be brittle. Have a say in things, you might just see.

What is this that befouls our mood? Are we ready for a chance? Is this what we seek? I am one to wonder at the ripeness of things. And here, where the measure is of the sandstone, and what is left is of the nestling, we find ourselves anew.

Constancy, and a repour that delineates. There are things here we don't understand, but must engage with. There is a semblance of normalcy, but what of it? We will come again, and know things to be in their right place.

Cobwebs – dusted. Confirmation, and roundabouts. There is nothing more than this. Nothing more in the show. We come for the cause, and know ourselves to be wounded. But what is at issue is that which guides us. We will let it.

What is the case of it? Small, but with frills? I am one to believe in great things, and here, where my heart resides, I skimp on nothing that would excite. Do not leave me opinionated, I fear for the laughter – but have nothing left.

Sources of joy, sources of pleasure. I know what sings, and what harks. We hark, for simpler things – more that is encouraging of the times. Here we go – one, two three; and there we go, a roundness of indifference.

Come splashing in, there is nothing to it. And then, like figurines, we harness the realm, and see what can be seen. We fight, but lay down our weapons for the shear sport of it – and then, like May, it sprinkles like a dove.

Much is like the rest. Much is here to stay. Much is in the wind. I will have nothing more to say, nothing more to say, except this – 'I will hear until the day I die.' And in that there is motion, and in that there is heart. We will transpire.

Never before have the sounds of so much been so enshrined in forever. And then, without a thought, without nous nor incumbency, a truth settles in vaster realms, and gives a glare at all. We have won. We have won.

Notwithstanding anything, we must all endeavour to display our right minds in times of diligence, times of sorrow. And then, a remembering trick – we have seen it all, time and time again. There are flares that ignite, and flares that cause darkness. Yes.

Constant motion – that is what we need, and what we have. There is nothing, when we look, that we don't have. All we must do is look, and lo it is found. Never distrust the embers of time, they are here for us.

Vacant to the touch, we see ourselves in staunch disregard to the levity of all things. Much is right, and much is left, and all that will be is here. We do not descend here, only float up, and let ourselves catch on the line of it.

Seeming like a summer sun, but not buying the trappings. I am one to sail through the mist – I am one to see things anew. I have felt sure in things, so have not reneged. I am here like never before. I am here.

What is this thing we have believed in? It is all of us, combined, and weeping. What is the travesty we thought had gone, but was just below the surface? And here, where our footsteps come briefly, a new step, to welcome the old.

Come, let us not fix ourselves to the mast – the squall comes, but we are ready. The squall beckons, but we have no fear. Do not reckon each one of us together. Long is our way, long is the meeting of things to come. We are ready.

Hanging on to the distance. We love this where it comes to. And then, like a wind in meditation, we see more than we ever have. Catching the fibres as they fall. Being menaced by good taste. We shall do it again.

Gleaning something more, and having it shine. What we have left is something of a mystique. And then, like rubber on the tarmac, we see our chosen direction. And now without a blink, we are there.

A mission to see things straight. A confidence to align things, due north. And then, like a blizzard near the sea, our heart beats, beats in time – in time to what? In time to all things; all things that beat in similar fashion.

Aspiring towards the sunset, towards the dawn. What is left of us, now that we have arrived? What is the sand between our toes? What is the wind amongst our hair? We have gathered, but for what? We will have mirth, but when?

Nestled in close, there is a way to be. Being not scared of embers in the dark. I have found a way through the charm and the abyss. I have sensed what is to come. And then, like a firebrand in full light – we have it.

A lark we see ourselves as – a vice-royal accompaniment. And here we change guard, guard of the ruse. Come now, sense is all pervading. This should be something to work towards. We have it in sight.

Amongst the rubble, we look out. And here, where the sun does not shine, a masquerade goes on, one that hides no blemish. I think I see Byron, in all his finery. It is like a swim in the sea – let us laugh.

Verisimilitude, and what is left. I will bargain a new price – one that no seal bonds, nor any heal sews. Come now, what we love, we can only have in spits and spurts. What is here, is never now. What is now, is the life of it.

 I will only believe one thing – the stars give a maddening waltz. But what is nonsensical to us, is not so to the bereaved. Not so to anyone. Not so to this or that redemption. Be in line with what comes. We will wander.

Let us listen – listen to the clouds. We are wanting to be here – like never before. There are chances that dispel the mist, and chances that do not. Seeth in wonder, we come for you. But then, speak of what you like, stances are here to be filled.

Further into the rain, we seem more acclimatised than before. But here, where the sand does not tarry, there seems a nice place to find rest. We were questioning where to go next, but have found our way. This much is sure.

Languishing in the middle of things, we are apt to say something to the night sky. But what good can a verbal display do to end the reunion of souls as they leave in perplexed affection. We will see them again.

And here, like a wastrel, like a dalliance that does not sing; here can only be what may. I am testing the waters, and that which I find pleases me, like a test to the departed, like a mesmerising that only dismisses. We will find ourselves.

And there, in the howling wind, something great appears. It is something we have not seen in a millennium. But what of its cause? What of its truncated rhythm? We have seen that before. I will never again see the likes of it, though. We will trail.

Much is said of the passage of regard. Much is said of its elegance. Much is remembered to this day, to this day of its grand intersection with the stars. I know you are something to be still by – but what of this? What of this?

So much for the white of it, we will gather new gowns to sew, new wilds to reap. And then, like a lurch in the darkness, there comes a sweeping through the vastness. We are here, here where we want to be. We know no other way.

What I once heard, was my heart, beating, beating afresh. I was on the coast, and there we have it- the sound was the same. The sound was the same. I will not linger; fingernails have a knack of breaking.

There is a crest, one amongst it all, that knows no flurry, nor time to rest. Come now, alleviate your suffering, such that you have time to fall. There is here, something small, that grows upon command. Such is the feeling of our journey.

And then, like an alarm clock at 12, there is a time to right the ship, and have as your blast the somnolence of a power from some other place. It is here we offer you this. Do you fend, or do you give way? – We shall see.

Transpiring, and in line. The feeling we once felt cannot hold us. We listen, but where is the moisture? Come now, seek remission in the heart. There are travesties we just cannot capture.

And when we cry, the tears that we shed are not of this earth. They are from the land of the unheard. And here, the simplicity of what we seek is enough to fill a bowl of neverness – right to the top.

Below, there is a sign. Its station is to wallow – but when the time is right, and everything is perfectly aligned, a sense of relief, and all the collar will seek. Much to digress – much to call to salience of things. Much.

And now we see before us, love and all its demise. Come along for the ride, things are looking towards the sky, and in proportion to what we seek. I love this part of things, where furniture is re-arranged, and tasks are here for handling.

Come with us, says the happenstance, there is a new insistence, a new instance that alters the way. Come, we are obliged to assimilate stores of the renowned – into each and every condition. Do not list, the sea is rough.

And again, I say, believe in the sea, believe in the heart, believe in their hearing, it is not to be lost. Rather, it is found, it is here, it is not squandered – it is a realm, the encounters all, that partakes in winter water. Have this, I ask of you.

And now, with a long delay – something special, to the hills, and valleys, of this world. There is a driving force that whispers in-absentia, that forgets itself in the renegade fury, and that says, simply, I will not go.

A caustic wand that drives no belonging, something that we herald as cheap, but stills in wonderment and transpiring grace. I am the one to sing its praises, because in this realm, longitude and latitude hear no mirth. Yes.

Like a magic full of pride, sustenance betides us. And then pulling back, there comes a thinness to life that we hope will never pass. But what of the slowness of our walk? Distances never matter, only backwards motion.

Inside the workings of it, we see ourselves in splinters of light. And here, where there is no way out, we find more than enough to keep us company. Distractions are awry, but what we see cannot be faulted.

I have once or twice faded into bloom. And here, where no one has been, I sit and write myself anew. Much of what is next could fill a volume or two, or something else besides. What is this I hear you ask? It is more than we can comprehend.

Rolling, with wisps, with tundra in check, there are places to go, places to be. And now, despite ourselves, we linger by the grave, and know our grace to be beguiling. Do not fear, hundreds of us pass this way every day.

Our feet are pressed in bars of tenderness. What is left, has a science to it. And now, a longevity to listen to, passes this way. Co-mingle certain senses prevail in certain circumstances. This much can be said.

Gushing, and being loud. Seeing what comes next. Being what the sea wants, and what we hold most dear. There is a sink hole here, but we do not ingrain our steps. What we fancy to do, is drive away, one fashion at a time.

Lots to do, some say nothing, some say all. There can be tension left after this. What is more, is that tendrils of life that hurry as things swimming in water, will never find themselves a place to migrate towards. That much is clear.

Something like this has come to the fray. We fight, but fight for what? It is all in us, and all about spilling from the sides. There is like a festooned love that has a palace of share intwined through and through.

And now, looking backwards, somewhere else
encumbers the scene. There is like a new found
land, one that militates against refinement, and all
its splendour. There is something to be sought
here – and something to be placated.

What was once a size apart, is now the
semblance of things to come. Be tried and tested,
and all that is left will be yours. Afterwards – after
this – a place of experience, one that fills. We will
come.

A laughter emanates from the room. Something
we didn't expect. And now, like a sort of ancient
ritual, life comes spiralling down through the roof.
And then, despite it all, we love what we have
been given.

There is a sense in which the noise of bicycles
stems from the heart. And here, where we never
knew when to go, and when to stay, there is a
package or us, lounging in mid-air. We will reckon
when it is time to open it.

A vastness, that lingers out of time. A belief that
worries about nothing. There is space in the forest
to hear the bastion cry. And then, like now, a force
to things that has as its council a nebulous kind of
life. We will not falter.

Wishing for the daylight. A genuine attempt at all.
What is here, is not there. What is there is
roundabouts. Come and be the soldier in a
soldier's garb. But bring no weapons, there will be
no fighting – maybe a tear to catch.

Hard lived, and hard read – bistros of
complacency. Never receding, only delivering –
there is nought to do here but deliver – what is fun
and fashion to us? We loved our finding that came
to the line. But what is that? We will see.

A claustrophobia that only remits. What is now
pure, and hardly settled on. Much is said here,
much delayed. I am sure of one thing – life
straddles the confines of this or that maelstrom.
We will revel in all of it.

Above, as below, fires that do not weep. Stars that
remain motionless in a sky that is set for
breathing. Come here for a moment, treasures
dispatch after the consolidation of light. Set
yourself for the motion.

Sensations that do not whimper. In style, there is
no comparison. In wit, not a travesty to be seen.
The land within – the great unexplored expanse.
There is now time to reflect upon the day.

I have seen many things – one thing I haven't is you. But that is okay, paces are made for walking, and the dishevelled makes us recline. We have found now a trail through the mud and water – such that now we see.

Chapter 3.

Soliloquy and the depth of it. We know our shores,
but what of our remainder? The transference of
energies is here. What is white paints itself blue.
What is now, comes in bags of simplicity. Do not
follow yourself around corners – that will not
suffice. In adjusting, we have found our true edge.
Do not blister, the times are not here. There is a
misanthrope, who harks no sound. Tell me
something I would like to hear. Your majesty, do
you set the parlance?

Much in store, much in store for life itself. There is
a commiseration to uphold, and we will do so. And
then, like a fish on the golden-blue waters, we will
wish ourselves away, until there is nothing more.
Come now, a sequence of events holds us in
sway. But that is not enough to curtail the embers
nor the sparks of a world on fire. Believe in the
wonder of it, it will only cast. But cast what? That
which is most adhered to the wind. But is that
enough? I sincerely hope so.

To harvest what is left. This is what we are doing
here. But what we are not doing, is letting things
settle, to all the vibe of station. Be a hardship, and
nations will abide you. Count on nothing but the
thoughts of tailors, and the residue of something
new will have its country to absolve. Much now
rests on the concurrent amusement of daffodils –
stems above the rest. I will find a new way to stay,

and flay, but not betray. We listen, and our coughs are loud. Be boisterous – it will suit.

Attention, is only a path towards something else. What is this but the substance of our meal? What is this, but the nomenclature of what is left? We see ourselves in autumn dress, and know the finding of swept up leaves to be a blessing and not a curse. Be that as it may, we will not be dismissive, of ways to go, or undulations to travel. I will only say this – temptations are the life, but what you should know is that bliss always comes with a hurdle. Remember that, and all will be fine.

There is a gap where my heart once was. In its place the sea pulses, and knows no respite. There is a time for all that frolics, and all that is new. Be the masthead, and what you will see is a vast coastline, that lingers in sempiternal array. Never before have we seen the lanyards keep pace. I know of nothing else that will quell the notions of the clouds. I can write – but can I live? We will have to rest our shores on firmer sands. This much we can do.

There are thousands of ways to reel in the labyrinth. And in this, there is one that stands out. Prick your ears, find a stethoscope – travel down to the coast. Listen to your heart, listen to the sea, and what's more, hear their similarities. There is time to do this all-in-one day. But don't dismiss the results – it is a certainty they will surprise. We cast a shadow, in time to the chosen few. But what we say, is nothing beyond our play. Mischief is a salamander, ripe for the solstice.

There is a lot to be lost, here in the neverlands – but much to be gained. I have felt remorse at the tug of a jumper – at the tug of its sleeve. I know what comes with simple motions, and simple hearts. An echo that hears only itself. A sea that pounds for you. I am one to situate my life without the sounds of togetherness, without the bounds of love. There will be a new way to be – one without the curfew or the wax. This is how we know – we will see.

Longing through the sand, and coming through in wisps of grey. There removes from the daylight all that could be. But what is left? Much, and much about. We will gather ourselves for wanting, and the aridity of the journey. We must be fond of this, fond of the way we seek. It drags us onwards, and through, and then besides. We cannot even see the ramparts that contain us. But that is fine, as long as our soul is strong, and the fibres of our way even stronger.

We have never missed a beat. In this, there is a chance to value the day for all it is worth. And now, things are spread, and things are there. I know something else to – what we see in the dawn, is more than we can elucidate, in this or that turn. There is a price to pay for beauty, and we will pay it. And then, the noise we all make descends from places unknown, and sends our bones a brittle. Do not come, the sands will not hold us.

There is something we don't understand in all of this, and that is like a rising tide, things will come and go. The mainstay of the closing, that holds its breath for too long – like that, and stronger still. We will not submit. For any world, for any part-world. There is a moisture in the air here. We can taste it. I will tell you only once, and then not for forever. Classical pains in an age of apogees. Come now, we can never lose faith. That much is clear.

Thanking all who are present. Being wise to the surrounds. I am here, where forests lurk. I am here where the tests come in stages. There will never again be a way like this. I have plunged into it – the best I can. If I have erred, I have done so for beauty. If I have travelled, I have done so with heart. But what of it? What of the rind, and the touchstone? What of our forebears, and their song? We will mark our steps on greater wings, and have as our annulment, more to do.

When the fire of our lives departs, what is left is the sanguine and the beach. Never before have things meant so much. Never before have the sides of it been so acclimatised. I am here to tell a story, one that has no end. I hope your ears are for hearing. I hope your hearts are for the listening. I saw someone today I hadn't seen for a while – like the clouds, full of life. And like clouds, simply moving. There will be nothing like this again.

And then, like a raging that doesn't cease, untold dominions unfold in gusto. I will sing to you, until nothing is left. Until that time has diminished – until that time – we will rush for the exit, and know things to be great. Have we that in us? Have we the smart of the journey? Do things not ride in a certain fashion? – Swing in a certain fashion? We know, but do they? What is this like, that tantalises so? There will only be time to see the birds fly, and that is all.

 First of all – things don't fit. And when they do, they crumble. Never mind the land-wash, something that comes to a halt in grand succession. There is time here to witness the sands as they travel in undulating plateaus, a sight that every marksman salutes. And then, as in now, there is a rumbling, one we would rather not hear. We hear it, though, to our distress. And then like magic – to our merriment. There is a face here, one that says – yes, time. And we stare.

I know my way. It is like steel, like ice. And then, like a sense of what is to come - it is strong, and without feeling. It measures itself in ardent passions, and fallen wishes. We must not follow, we must only be the chosen, to listen to the entree, and reciprocate in mind, and in fashion. I will live here, until living is no more. What more can be said? What more can be tempered? There is a nothingness here, a tribesman who elects to stay and support. Study well.

What did we lose? But nothing. What did we say? But all. And then like a withstanding shadow, we come in full light. But what do we say (refrain)? The tempest marches on. We know it is syncopated, and in need. Come now, we love what we see. We love what we see, and what we feel. This is best. But what of the encumbered, those in shells of grief, and partitions of gold. Never whisper, only in times of sparseness. We will come - and then?

Tantalising, and with effort, we see ourselves fly. But what of the night? Does she turn - turn in shades of travesty. There is something not to be missed. But what is that? We don't know – all we know, is that the barriers of acceptance, are like the furtherance we never heard. Do not overlap, the distance here relates to us as we are finding trails in the heart. I am like the forlorn, but I have a wondering in me that shouldn't be. I will walk – walk like never before.

A lost visage – oh well. What we have come for, is the lesson of the stream. But then, like a pulse in the twilight – things come, and things dread. I have thought nothing more of things astray, but have not determined their lineage. It is not a farce, but a well-earned break. What is left is hard to see. But we limit ourselves to a farthing a notice. What of this, we don't know. But what we do know, is in fenced and tired ways, we begin once again. We have a plan.

Thinking a lot, all the time – thoughts become their own life. And then, like something in the middle, a carriage to carries the load. I am one to believe in things. I stop and start, and go forward where I can. There is something magical about this, and it stoops as it transforms. I will come again – if only to see things aright. I have never known things like this. Believe in the strength. It is something mesmerising – something great. I will never cease – never.

Half listening – I hear something. It is the sea. But what next – I rest my palm to my chest. There is here something deep. But where is the source? And that to has a feeling. I long for the chase, but heavy in its embrace. And now, without the slightest care – a trick. One that pleases as it unwinds. I have felt this before, a long-time ago. But in the stillness, a sense of well-being. There will come a time for things to be, and then we will know - this much is certain.

Much will remain. Much will be still. I know now, there is much in me, much that drives. And here, where the belief in all things surpasses itself, there will be time to spend alone. But what is this (already here)? And now a fusion of lives, that come in thick halves. I will see again – before you know it – and then a raft unto the sea. Do you hear it? A heart beating. Do you hear it? We come in waves to see this. And then, like this in a rough way round – we will find it.

I will listen closely – more closely than ever before. But when I am done – this, and this alone. I knew our departure would be fraught, but that is in the weave of things. I should have known better than to rake the grass before your arrival. And now, and now and then, a lopsided delivery, that has as its mark more of the sympathy, and less of tears in the night. There will be nothing left.

There is a bitter taste in this mouth. It harbours no ill-will. But that is okay. I sense something intangible, more than before. I know that without the fight, things would be stationary. And here, where the languishing of fire-flies denies, a new found land, that engages us in new ways. I think it is here, where we can find our lives again. But what is wrong with now? What is wrong with the journey? It labours, but for what? It labours, but for whom? We will never know.

And when everything is settled, much time for rest. We have not seen things like these in a lifetime. Please be what the sand sees. Please be what we never thought possible. I think, in line with the suits of old, we have formed a newly invented raft, such that, when we arrive, we do so with aplomb. What is that you seek? A fanfare? We will see to that. And when we have, much in the way of rejoicing. I know this will not hurt, on the contrary – pleasure awaits.

A bucking, we never had observed before. And when time renounced all its needs, there was one that remained. And that one, was something special. Something we saw only in silhouette. And now, without comfort or ease – without lifting nor pulling – we see ourselves fly, higher than the sparkling mass, on ten-folds of shoring ebullience. There is something that has a mould to it that will not render, or see fit. And this is it. We have come full circle.

And now, with nothing more than a quizzical stare, and seating to unnerve, we are left with something more – something more to miss a beat by. What do we say to this, oh brow beaten one? Where is the rejoinder? I am pithy in the mode, but what of in dimension? Solid, and desiring. There is nothing left – of our ease, of our sound, of what we thought best. I know this will hurt – but let us have the conversation, and then we will know what intrigues us so.

The sunlight parts, as we drive into park. We are at the university, where I once graduated. The clouds ripple, as the sound of sandwiches never swims. We are all here to sample the past, and indeed know it to be fine. What we did here will last. What we did here will find a care – in-between amusings and the rest. What have we found here? What have we seen here, but our former selves, that beckon a thing; a thing unknown, or untold.

To begin, again. Now, without applause, or whispers from any quarters, a new way has descended. But from where, from whom? From the past, from the present, from the future? Do we see it in the rhythm of life? Do we cancel what we love for it? There can be no other dimension to it. And here, where rope and tinder exaggerate our feeling, so too does the meanness of the journey. We will not have it. No, we will not have it – I am adamant in that, And I shall remain so.

What do the clouds do to upset us? What does the closer fusion of love and hate bestow on the unwary? There is something more here – something we don't yet quite understand. But we are willing to wait, to see intrusive outcomes in abeyance. What is left? What can be said? I know of no other, comparable acclimatising. But here, where life is a passing show, we will say a good guidance to what is called for, and yes to the daylight.

Water course, absolving no other. We sing, but
what for? We dance, but in inclination for what? I
have never known a swim more invigorating. What
is left of the sky is enough to fill a boat. But then,
who wouldn't. A fable, one that has us all aghast,
belittled, but never mistaken. Always beholden to
someone, or something. Catching a new sense of
old words. There can never be anything more
attuned than this. We will ride.

Vexatious and alive. Vexatious and teaming with
life. I never saw something so enamoured by life.
And then, something we need to do – immerse
ourselves in wonder. How deep? As deep as it
goes. How long for? – The remainder. How far? –
For the distance. And this is something in
splendour – wonder and its derivatives. We will
have fun here, these sands and I. Do not test our
strength with the tricks of swanning through, and
above.

This spot is sacrosanct to all who see themselves
as wandering. It is here, where the fallen and the
lost come to gather. And so, where the moisture
doesn't rise a minute of life, there comes a new
sense to old charms. Be here, we love the arms
around us, and the telling of winter stories, stories
that warm as they cover. I know there is nothing in
the void of it, but I wish to be sure. And that I am.
Come now, stories are all we need. And we will
have them.

Coming through in stages, we wade in the mist like through a thick soup. And then, time cannot see us. And the reverie we seek has no hands to catch. And now, like a levity that holds all it can, there is peace, and calm, and a certain solace. I know, now, of no other way. This is where we come from, and this is where we will return. There is like a smoothing over inequalities, and a sense to remove all disdain. What have we left, but what was given to us?

A mingling that ripens the door. Some such thing that opens our eyes. We now see ourselves covered in snow. But what is the temperature outside? What is it that drags us on? We have every bit of what we need. But what is that? You will see. But what is that? On the contrary, what is this? Brandishing a keepsake. What is this in your hand – more than we could imagine. Do not worry yourself now – the times are changing – if not for good then close to it.

Bringing with us more of the same. There is a chosen smile that greets. Have you your say? And then, either way, diminish in circles. But then, in aggrandizing refrain, much that will suit. Come and be for the folly of it. Come and be for the way it turns. And then, like a fountain that herds no cattle – we listen again, like the wand that hurts no soul, and the pitching of summer residue. We will eek a life out here, and know it to be one of pleasure. Do not hold on – maybe with one hand.

Gosh, and bother. Which way to turn? Which way to go next? I have known a thousand people. But as of late, none. I have known a thousand people, and as of late none. There must be something to catch on, to see them all again. There is a future here, but which one? See ourselves fly again, and float down to earth. See this thing called earth, and then in knowing rush at life. We cannot resist, nor take our turn. We feel for nothing else.

There is a cleansing motion that recites in the yard something of the tree. And then, like the asp, a sense of the wonder of it. Do not still yourself, there is much to do. And here where venom is young, a sort of sortie that uplifts despite itself. There is a wing that knows only the ground. And here, there comes the dimensions of sight. I can see this far, and this far only. Whatever your dimensions, we need your help. Will you give it?

The clouds move slowly – but what doesn't is our hearts. We can thank them for that. But now, for the challenge of the sea. How wide in the widest ocean? How deep the deepest sea? And the heart. How large the largest heart? How strong the strongest? There is now a length to see unfold, and we will see it. There is a mixture here, of sorts, that contains all that is. We will follow it, until time itself ceases. The moisture here in the air resonates with our larger journey.

Greetings from all that sustains us. Greetings from the very fibre of things. Greetings from what comes next. Greetings from the arc of life. We are famished, but strong. Strong but heartened. Desiring, but what suffices, will do. I am here, like never before. I am here, beside the gravestone. I run, but prefer to walk. I see life, envisioned from afar. There is like a siesta in the afternoon – will you come? I hope so.

Much intensity – much laughter. This is the way it should be. Without the knives nor the stakes, or any of that which brings us down. There is time to hear things aright. But what is that which keeps us going? I don't know. But what I do know is that the swing that brought us here is something that can never stop. But what of the fencing off of life? What of the challenge of the night? There is much to see here, and much to do. We will envision something more.

There is more to this than it seems. What is that, I hear you ask? I am unsure. But what I do know is that if one conquers the mind, much ensues. But that is a rough guide only. The sky – the clouds – the horizon – the twilight – and all things. There is a roughness where the bold sit. It is the world. There is much to do around these partitions. And when we counter ourselves against the gate of life, somehow, and in some way, things get better. There lies a truth.

Having something more to say. Having something more to do. There is a window that looks out onto an ancient sea. And it is here where we find ourselves. Rolling, pulsing, converging. And now like something that comes with the rain, a new dance, that has as its domain, melancholia. We wait for the feelings, and without a second to lose, we have them. As we do a sort of finality in the wind. We gush, and pout, and finally find. This is what we have come for.

Chapter 4.

Whispering, in time to the chosen few. There is a lingering we are foretold of, that carries with it much needed supplies. And then like the sand of a thousand beaches, we come and revel, such that our revelling lasts the journey.

A tender point, right in the middle of things. Right out of the corner of our eyes. There is much to be said, and much to be told in different ways. And here (hear) there will be gatherings, of this or that mode.

A hollowed-out canoe, raging down the raging river. What was once in line, is now in check. We hurry from the canoe and reach firm ground. We get back in, and ride the boisterous water all the way to calmer banks.

Cascading, and all through. Warming for the challenge. There is time – time to wait. Time to be, time to see. With water behind our ears, and our hearts wrapped in tears – we will come with fears (to be abandoned).

Wall of ice – wall of fire. There are petitions in the sand, that only rub on wood. Come and see us, we are here for you. And then, like a place we have hardly been to, moisture, and the semblance of the journey.

Wailing, and gnashing. Life confronts us. We do not move. What we do, though, is something special. We find a sense amongst it. And then, like chiselled road, we come. Like a distance that has no eloping. Here we are.

Without forcing, only to prise – what we have is a solid form. The form is one of attendance, that we see in the foyer. There is now a show, one that depicts the wholesome and the glad. What is that? We will see.

Forming an opinion, one we should do to carry on. Carry on the ship, or as we please. Witnessing the wind blow as hard as it gets. We are there for retribution, and our namesake. Not to mention the colours of yore.

Developing a rheumatism, and watching it fade. Seeing things straight for the first time. Believing, but not being entangled. Sighing for more. Being askew, but never minding. Being at work, and never stopping.

Distance, and feeling. At home, and despite. We live, and grow, around the template of the heart. And then, festivities, and much more to come.

Maybe tempered, but still to please. We have won a victory against the night.

And now, we will believe, in the semblance of the centre piece, and all that is through. I have known treasures alongside the sea, and I have felt all that is. I cannot stand the wiring in this place. I look on, and there is respite.

Come now, what do you say? What have you seen in amongst it? Much desire, a buoyancy. There is like a ruined castle here, ancient. I have let you go, to do as you wish. Buoyancy, and the mode of miles.

A desperation in the wind. More calling for air. We swim, but what of the cost? There is sand, but we can move it. There is a feeling buried deep, but dig we do not. And then, we carry ourselves forward – much to do, much to say.

Further than the wind – further than the shore. I see myself wading through shallow pools. And here, where my heart gives way, I know that things are precious. There is now a time for reflection, and a time for knowledge.

A little-known fact has come alive. We see it, but do we touch it? There is a silence here, one that doesn't beckon. Believe in the thorough-fare, things will temper. Now is the wellspring, just as time is the boon.

Constantly surprising – there is a way forward. And the possibilities – welling up. Where are my dreams today? We come through, and then know our place. White-song, there is a lamentation.

Aloft, and with heart. There comes a challenge, which we see, and see off. There are motions, despite. There is movement, and acclimatising to say. We find Faust, and read it at our leisure. There is always time for this.

There is a place – beyond all places. There is a time, that has only itself to fashion. And here, where we all come, there lies no waste, a general meaning to be, but no fathoming to distance any remonstrations. We will find it again.

Much can be said of the wanting mass. Much can be said of the treasure in silk. Much is known of all that is. But what is not known, is how? And, why this? We circumnavigate the world, searching, but we see ourselves aloof. We will walk.

And now, with a taciturn smile, we come to that point where we must surmise. And here we do. But what of the fabric of the tension of it? We are

here not to gather, so we won't. We are here not
to sell delights, so we won't
We harvest, but what of its ilk? – We line the
roads, but how far can we see? I am one to tempt
the bastions of their very foundations. Do not
blaze on silt, we come for more than this. There is
now a difference between this and that. We will
sway.

What is this thing called life? We sense long in the
incubation. Travels, and inspirations. Much travel,
and much inspiration. Formidable, and
unhindered. Do we cause it all – some. But what is
that we seek out of all this?

Conscious, and alone. We find time to sit and be.
And here, where our backs are in fact arched, we
settle our ancient scores, and then, know how to
talk. Believing in the simplicity of it, we tend to our
thoughts, and know something of them.

Gathering steam – it is like a nursery rhyme –
gathering steam, we find the tempest has abated.
But what of this? - equally in transit. Much
insistence, insistence that we seek. And then a
likened satellite, one that bores in deep. Yes, we
will.

Naming, and being cursed. Fairing little better, but
holding on. There is a diamond that does only
shine for us – but what is it for? What does its

shine entail? We know much, but of this? Included in the run of it. We are near.

Stellar, and new. Stellar, and around. Stellar – what was that? We include in our lives more than is enough. We are of heart and soul and sea. We hear it all – one thing after the next. But where is our dreaming, our dreaming state? We will see.

Lifting, and seeing through. Seeing through, and being surprised. A mish-mash of colours that uplifts. Do not bend in the wind, it will only break you. Heaving, despite, and having a weight lifted.

There is much to see – much to do. With this in mind, it would be laboursome - but then, without thought of ourselves and our station – we launch into work instead. There are joys here, and painted halls – is this what we seek? We will know.

There is a sense we all have, that the horizon is sacrosanct, that what believes itself to be in the marrow, is nothing other than the mischief of this fight to the next. We all must take instruction. But here? Yes indeed.

Are we to sow the seeds of yore, or are we to sail our ships through straights undaunted? We unveil our most precious insight, and see it tether. But what of the now? We may never know. What we think, goes.

And then, like a thought betokened, we leave our visage at the water's edge. Do not speak in hums, there is a reason for it. Here, where our lungs breathe red air, a manifesto of life springs, like the surface of a breeze.

Catching the mezzanine before it falls, we see ourselves in retrograde motion. Is that what there is, life amongst the things that fall? And now, believing again, we decide where we will go. That is one thing we can be sure of.

What is this we see? Is it the road, or the shoreline? Can we ever be sure of which. I sing to you, only because the depth of things is advantageous to my life. Be here, so that things will not turn, turn in a roundabout way.

What can only be said, must be seen as intangible. What there is, is the soap on winter barriers. We will believe in chance, until there is no more. And then, like a cradle before the moon – mystique, and adventure.

There is a looking glass, that sees right through to the bottom of souls. And in this glass, there is no formidable opponent, no dare I say life, no incendiary aplomb. What we see is pure and simple. Much to our delight.

And now for the report – we sound our lives on things which never beckon. We sound our lives on the space between egg-shells. What is never enough is the sound itself. We come, and are forgiven.

Minute by minute – hour by hour. We preclude what we see and hear. And we come back down to the resonating board, that treasures all we know. Do not fend off, there is no time. We will fight the undeniable – and here find our leisure.

There was never once we shirked. And here, where life transmutes into day, we find a fellow traveller singing the same song he always has. And then again, the beholden and the wit come to play - and then? Indeed

Flash, and through. Having an alignment, and never worrying. I will come for you out of the blue, and see ourselves in-potentia. I will never stop, not for this, not for that. We will build a mound in honour of the day.

There is a festivity at the bottom of the hill. We see it, and are intrigued. What is now, is like grace. What is then, is like ice. Too cold to touch. And

then like a landfall, we moisten our lips, and say –
'Who's who?'

And then, we liken our gaze to a piece of steel, as
it comes, and as it is ready. There is patience
here, and like-minded souls. And here where the
journey meets the sea, tenacity, and the hearing
of something special.

Much that comes with us. Much that second
guesses. Much that has the wind for
companionship. Be true and linger. Be the one
never to subside. Only daring is in order. Dare,
and be fresh. Be fresh and wander.

A distance that matters. Weaving in and out of the
night. Something tangible, which guides the way.
A heart that rolls. A sea that is heard. What makes
this reality? – only us. There can be no other way.

Considerable aplomb. Nearing elation, we check
where we are. And then, like a whisper from a
stranger – we walk that bit harder. There is more
to this than we think. It comes into vision.

Any time for the winding? We will once again
dance, dance like a word has a meaning. There is
the intractable – we must not forget. Love and life,
and the bridge in-between. Come now, we must
only convey.

A load hauls forward. We find a way to accompany what is there. And then, like the trees of flight, we flood down in torrents, and then in sheets, and then in cosmopolitan dreams. We will never ask again.

What is this, that is missing? Is it our hearts – minding themselves? Is it the sea – bold enough? We launch right into things, as they are. Belief and the wonder of it. We know what to do next.

Holding on, we sample the refrain. And know that life is the sort of thing that has as its base all the tribulations of the land. We know now what is to come – we have tempered the stance. Forever in line to the notion of it. There we have it.

Reaching for something different. There is a place for that here. And then, like a range that never sleeps, a new fashion that believes in itself. Caustic and awake, things treasure in the folds of fabric. We will come.

Commit to nothing. Commit only to the motion of the sea. And then, like a day-dream, it comes. All the places, all the sounds, all the direct courses of action – here and now and through and beyond. It will be.

Silence – but what of it? Who comes to place?
Who is in the mould? What withers, until withering
replenishes. What have we now, that time lingers?
There is more than we can say. There will be time.

Much in line – much to say. Much that does not,
but much that does. We will rinse our senses, and
hear the goading force bring itself unto time again.
We have nothing to give, except our hearts, which
are not constrained. Life, yes.

Considering things lately, there is a nuance to its
temporality. We love what we do, but the
sequence firms. Minor, this is what we say. There
is a time for all plays. Time for the management of
wit, and the station of surprise.

All dressed in white, and looking like an honour
bestowed. What have we as a happenstance?
There is time to be – we must. There is time to
see. We must not arrange. The sea will not let us
– but our hearts will. There is no complaining.

Harking back, there is no room. Salacious and
determined. What have we thought, but all things?
What have we tailored, but the night? Put your ear
to the ground, you will hear it. We hear it, you will
to.

Willing, and wishing – selling and sending, masts and head pieces. There is no telling of what could eventuate. We will know something though, and that is like wonder, sounds and ports have life.

Causal chains, and recipes to find by. There is a new sense of awe to greet us. But what of the task at hand? It lingers by the night, and delivers the founding stone unto the building – what do we find? We can never part with it.

Science and reason, top down, down up. We have half the sense to breathe, and half again to drink the water. There is now a feeling like has never been, and never will be. What do we make of it - science and reason?

Passion and desire, which is greater? Passion and desire, the thumb is up. Passion and desire – much in store. I have never felt the pull of the dream, until I could see the score. There is not the wing of possibility to decide.

Capturing something special – leaving nothing on the dance floor. There is now a distance between what I love, and what I can see. But that is okay, necessity sweeps all before us. But before it does, more of what brings us.

There is now more life than we thought.
Adjustments and foreseeing. Considerable souls
away. And then, like a beating heart near the sea,
away our life goes. There were times in-between,
when we never thought this possible. But now!

A feeling after the time, a silence, that rings true
through the world. Have the moisture dry, and the
well-being welled up. And then like that, the noise
of the carriage way diminishes, and sleep comes
in turn. We have wandered.

Certainly, here to stay, never here to go.
Wandering through the maladroit, we linger in our
own self-directed maze. What have the hills to
say? What is denser than the fibres of it all? We
are there now – we are there.

There can't be any more than this. The reaching
mass clambers over the hedge and belief, no
matter how strong. It is the beating of the heart
that ties things together. It is the beating that holds
sway. We beat, and we live. This much is true.

Ranging through, and not being held – that is the
goal. And it swims in costume and renaissance.
Have as nothing else the bind of it, and the
seesaw effect replenishes the goad. What is left of
it, is nothing short of all.

Swinging through, and around, and beyond. We find ourselves being polite, for a reason that all too much defies description. And then, like a song in the twilight, we callout, and know ourselves to be true.

And then, like mud in a reckoning bowl, we see the time of day, and know luck to be in wonderment. There comes a selfish desire, to do as we like, and do as we please. Come now, the sorts of things we do here will be palatable.

August and the light of it. The temptation to see things through. And then like a wayward sense through the night, morning comes. We see it, and know it to be strange. What can we say? Things will come.

Sensing the mist, we come full circle, and know that time will only bring what it wants. Do not be disturbed by this. For here, in the majesty of it all, new places to embark towards, new feathers to let float. We will unhinge, and be the desert.

Chapter 5.

There is now a bastion to uphold, one that does not slip. We see it mightily, and know that in the winter, the cold will not elope. There are people whom embark upon the way, but have as their base, the manufacturing of salt. And in that, joy, and the robustness of the journey. Give us the deadline, we will sing. We will be the mission, and the lost enclosure. Excitement, and the navigation of far reached places. There will always be the hand of the driver. This much is assured.

A cry in the night. A certain belatedness for the call. Are we believing, or are we settling in? Are we sleeping, or have we made up our minds? There is here a chance to be with windows as they look out over the sea. This much is combined with the gathered dust of a thousand years. Beat, beat, heart – you will win. What have you noticed, but all the rose petals in the world? What have you found, but this? There is always more to the story.

A fellowship of clouds that harbours all that is sweet. A belated treat that feels its way there. I know how this should go, but in that there is a catch. This is the way it goes – like this. And then a mast, one we cling to, and cannot let go of once we meet dry land. But that is okay, we each have our mast, and we each cling to it, no matter what. But it is here, that sands of the hour glass never shift. It is here, that we find ourselves again and again. We will not flinch.

Listening, intently, I see myself launching into life. And then, like a Hebridean stray, there comes a sound to belittle the mainstay. I will never really know what comes next. But what I do know, is that the time that is afforded to us is a monument, and a treat to be. Corners that heat, beat corners that street. And then like a renegade star, there bellows what is most in fashionable, and what is like nothing else at all, there is a further rolling that positions the sun as the moon.

Well-done-by, sisters of the meeting, of the tenacity to go by, of the wonder of it all. Dare I say, things which implode in our mouths are not the most common things to feel. And then, like writing through the sky, we head off in our chosen directions, and know things to be like they never were. What is now, is in autumn. What was then, was summer, what was past, was spring and winter. There comes a time for all things. We must not forget this.

Coming through in stages, we call out to ourselves from the roof tops, and know that the mission we have comes in cycles. We love this part of any adventure. The part where the walls slide in, and what is gone is only our hearts as our trepidation appears to wane. There is never anything like this. There is only this, as we lift our sight to get a

better vision. This is all that is. This is the
semblance of what is in life, and out of life. Come
and be bigger.

Feeling like the sand – difficult to curtail. And then,
in time to a melody we have never heard, a sense
of what is needed – needed by all of us. And now,
like a wisp of mist, something gathers, and we
know when to go and when to balloon back. I have
heard this place isn't much for runaways, but that
is okay, we don't run. I look up, and I see
something. It is us in our dotage years. What can
be more than that? All than that and more.

There is a treasure buried deep – how do we
discover its compartments? Through will, and the
fashioning of relief. There is nothing left to tell.
This is life, the fashioning of relief, and all that will
come to pass. We know a story, that comes in as
it pleases. There is a shield that belies the target
to renege, and all that we see. Come now, do
nothing that will hurt yourself. What is left is of the
nay-say, and what is left is of the dirt – but we can
make what we like of it. Yes.

There is a habit that tenders the likeness of the
sun. And that is walking. And when we walk, we
engage with the might of every firefly that has
been. Each time we walk we bend life that little bit
more, until, yes, it can bend no more. There is a
place for this, and it settles to arches and speedy
aplomb's. There is like a new good deal of

laughter. One that transmutes what is strong, and makes it manageable. We will be the ones with strength. We cannot be otherwise.

And when we come together, there will be a sound as has never been heard. It will be charged with temperance, and light - the fail-safe and the translucent. What we gather for is another matter. We gather for the sun. We gather for that which is left. We gather for the science of things, and the adumbration of what we see in the sky. There is equal measure here, and what cannot be contained. I have felt the barbs, now let us sing with great bravado.

Let the notion ring out. Let the tempest blast cry one more time. We are here, never to see things relate, nor time at the gate. There lingers one more time in the offing. We will not take it. The sense of it will only last for a period. And now, lingering through the way of it, a belief that strangers in the night are here to break down the barriers, and come through unscathed. What is left will not leave a mark, nor tarry gently. Come for the sky, it will help us acclimatise.

I have often thought, we can change things with our minds – any situation we find ourselves in, we can change – it is that simple. It is all about how much suffering we have been through beforehand. And then, like a catapult, change becomes a reality. All we have to do is tender ourselves low, and high we will become. Channelling what is in us becomes the norm. And we find ourselves with much to see, and much to do. That much is relied upon.

Mashing, and gnawing – giving credence to the light – being at once the invective, and the solo-reprieve. I come to vouch for. And in this there is a nation at liberty. In this, there rings a Corsican delivery. What we want, is the train that takes us there. What we want is all things together. What we want can no longer be fished from any sea. And then, like a treat made by your mother, we know where we stand. Could it be this? Could we stand again for hope?

For a reason I don't understand, there comes a simplicity to the night. And for another reason I don't understand, things are away that need to be tethered. I am at a loss to fathom each, but have as the chamber of my heart something we cannot catch, as a bluebird in the blue. What is this thing called love? What is this thing by-and-by? We have washed our hands of disinterest, but not of fate – all powerful and resigned. We will be still, and then our hearts will beat.

There is a message here in the sand. It reconvenes, and lasts the hour. We are forthright, and in need of a bridge. What of the lingering, and the namesake? What of the saleability? We will conquer, like never before. We will see the fibres of it, and know solace to be ours. And then, like a rainbow in evening light, we will touch God, and know friends to be prisoners in a strange land. Provoking of night. We will arch our backs, and know things to be well.

Aesthetically pleasing, and to the touch, a grace. Do we have so much as the fill that entrenches the soil, entrenches it deep, and with passion? We are reliable, and know the crescent to be so to. I am now in the right breeding for the approach, and here, have clear intent. I will not linger over glass, nor anything else, for that matter. I know of only one way through. And that is towards the entry, and through that way. There is a sound to hear – what is it? It is us, as we find ourselves.

There is a likeness to the stars. And here, where we come-to once again, there remains a template of ridges to fall against, and be over for. We must not wait, for anything, nor anyone. There is a light on the window pane – could it be any more beautiful? And sequins on the dial, remonstrating with the beauty, such is their courage, courage of life over death. And then, like a new-stand against an old warrior, we find ourself on pinions of flight – who knows when we will come down.

What is this Sunday of laughs? Do we tire of all things majestic? Do we flinch at all things bombastic? This meal, is entirely discerned through the five senses. And here, where the moisture of life abounds, we concern ourselves with what is out – outside and in the world – and not what is within, within us. There will be time for the table to be turned. But now, a juxtaposition, one that has as its forte the climes of being, the jungle of the heart – the space of the sea.

Fathoming through the debris of a heart that is not a mess. Being lucky, despite life. And then, a semblance of what is, and what is not. Do not tear away the keepsakes, they are for keeping, and not for leaving with. There is now a time for the rest of it, the rest of it to course. The sounds of invigoration spill forth, and know themselves to be tender, and away with things belatedly. And then, late in the day, a quiet that whispers sweet treats into all that is – Much to find.

Dragging what is left, we find ourselves tiring to the last. There are here now times for absorbing, and times for reminiscing, and times for having hold of what is best. I will keep going until going is no more. What can we feel, but the moon in flight? What can we find but the stratosphere in inertia? What can we find, but all that is? What is here, but timely events that save rather than hinder? There is precious little of all else. There is only time to keep us company. And we will keep.

Absolving of all and sundry, there is a mine to the heart that does not commit. And it is here, where the south wind blows its hardest, that the temper of the tempest rears, and the heart listens, but only stirs in unbelievable delights. I have felt this way before, and know that longing is not replete without guidance. There is a heading labelled 'south' that only visions itself in conundrums. And it is here that minds of marvel relate, and send this world spinning once again.

Harvesting through the mist, we long to see what we shall see. And then, in a Cartesian moment, we forget our world, and know there is no evil demon, just ourselves as we wade through. There is never any time to come back down to earth, and see the motion of the sea, as it ebbs and flows. What is this now, but all that is? What is this now, that contains all? We have never felt this way before. What is this place? What is this sound? The sound of things, the place of things.

Magisterial, and wandering through, there lies a time to be far gone, and a time to wish in the well. Never be too far gone – the world needs its anchor. And then, like a fire in the breach, worlds collide, and what is nascent becomes post and all of reality sinks in. There is never a time like this. There is only a time like this. We must always wish. As much as we can. Wish for the heart, wish for the sea, wish for all. We will not renege, nor dip our toe. That much is sure.

Much awake – awake and breathing still. Hard at heart, but breathing still. I will be one to settle old scores, to be the one to nestle in fibrous mass. There will much time for leisure, and pleasure and all things in due course. And then like a lightning bolt from beyond, sparks, and all the tribulations that have ever been seen. What is more, destinations, and all that comes. I have felt more of this that the world can concur. This much will fathom.

Forks in the road, splinters on the seat. We long for something more, something that can placate as well as heal. The turning circle of this ship defies. And then, with a gradient curve of insistent resolve, there comes around the sea a fashion such that the ringing in our ears must cease. We have nothing left to give. The festival of lights seems assured. Do not see things for the first time. The only time to do so is with the wind. And here, where we trade blows, dozens to speak of.

A sort of cavalcade, one that remembers where it is from. And then, like a sprite in the woods, a turning, that has us seeing red. I am like the daylight – I cannot see myself. What is laughable is the top note – but who cares; the fibres of this thing will never stop. There is a grimace where the sea once sang. And now, a feeling of quietude that sends the unflappable into raptures. Come now, no need for the snobbery. There is much to go around.

A fear we have that the crow is not now. Ruptured, and co-mingling. Sport, and the love of it. Mischief without cards. Seeing that takes its place. A mesmerising effect – something we will remember for future days, future years. Come now, the coalface is littered by the dimensions of heart. We have not withered, to say the least. There can only be the sage in all of us. Catching on, that is our job. Catching on. Yes. But we must say – life. It comes.

Gathering petals, the Faust in all of us says a belated 'time'. There is a mystery here, one that unfolds as it commutes. Do not shun, many mysteries are the most pleasing. I don't doubt you for a second. Come now, much style is garnished, much trial to the wind. I will have more of what can silence. In this, I hear the wind. In this the waves come flooding, much like before. In this a score to pertain. We will court the agenda, before it all begins.

Fast and secure – a tenacity that lingers. We will fight for once last glimpse. Glimpse of what? Of many things – paintings in an abandoned gallery in a deep forest – the grandeur of it all, as displayed by works of art, sculptures, installations, in that same gallery. There is much more to be said, much more to be shown. Much more to sense, and feel towards. There is a touch, one that we are familiar with. It comes in rays, that never stay. Committed to memory. We will not fast.

Conscious of the loss, we hear that our roundabouts are stretched to the screen of it. Do not prolong things, they are in hardship, and indecipherable. Much comes this way, and much to do has come to pass. We feel the remedy, as its sound revels in. I believe in the wildness of it. And here, where we assemble the lengths of it, there is a seat amongst the remainder. Have something small, and then once again believe in the crinkles of the mainstay. I have heard it said.

Coming through, with much haste. We then sit for a while, and know our place. It is here, where the sand does not turn. It is here, where the licentious unbridles its feathers, and knows that calm is the only way. Much to let go of, much to stay with. I have found things that go round, are not always the things for me. Mascarpone, delights – but what of the sensation of life? It can to. Feeling for the bliss, much comes with it. We will find a way.

And then, without respite, further appraisals form a ridge, that leaks only what comes next. Despite the ramblings of time, there exits something that cannot be contained. And it is here that layers of salt, layers of mist come together, to say – 'how' and then 'now'. But there is a trampoline in the way. But we will not fix it, it is the whereabouts of an awful dream. But we must dream. No matter how nightmarish, we will come again and again through it all to the end.

Lost in the grimace, sand comes too, to render all invectives dissolute. But what of the trenched and the nestled? What of these things we find here? Do we find the rounding of speech, and all that is treasured? Do we find ourselves, in comportment and in mode? There is a turbulence that should never tarry. There is a mode that truncates the distance of it. And here, I find this thing willing, despite the incursions that have nothing for life.

Like new, these things exalt the styling of ancient moats in ancient castles. I will not take longer that is commissioned. But how longer is that? Most of the night – ah phew. We expected as much. And here vengeful, and in need of a repositioning, things come, and things descend. I was in the making, and then things were made, and all that work just jumped high. What were we to do but celebrate? Missing corners, and the embrace of all things.

Come and be pleasant. Without this, the journey seems lonesome. It is not actually, but seems so. What is left of things, after our departure? Can we praise the watering can? Is this where our search ends? Is this where the noise of disinterest descends? Come now, what we need is the yoke to be vetted, and removed. Removed in this fashion, or that – it matters little. Come and be the story at the nearside. This will treat you well.

Descending, and feeling fine. Gaining in tropes, tropes that prefigure the dawn. Having as a land, a place that shouldn't be. Furthermore, having as a land, a place that can only be. What is the difference? None. Which is the tempest, and which is the night – or both? Which came first? Which tenders awnings bought from the outskirts? I am of the opinion that they can stay. A catch in the seam of things. A catch in that typecast that belittles the senses.

Condensed, and held in profusion. There is little that divides the heart from the sea. Both pulse, and have rhythm, both move us to act. Both have as the glands of a giving of health. Both can be clogged, but with work, can be relieved. And here where the midnight curfew rings still, the night and its remains, does work to rally us all. All we must do is gather ourselves for grace and livery, and what is more, the grand sweeping that holds us to everything.

Treasuring all that comes – believing that once again life will triumph. And then, like a god who knows which way, the semblance of tears, and the semblance of years. I have never felt so sure. There is a time, there is a wellspring, there is more than all of this. There is in the timbre of it a sensation that tracks as it harps, sees as it views, meanders through. Never before has the range of it been so aware. Come now, unshackle your intrepidness – single to fight back.

Much is said here – much that the forest knows
how to see. Much that our respective wellness
depends upon. And now, like tangles in the night,
a sense that things will be okay. And then,
standing on two feet, we see the arbour through
the mist, and know that things are there to be
solved. What is a problem without a solution?
What is the time of day without the need that
founds it? What is the lynchpin without the silence
that surrounds it? Much is said, much holds on.

Being astute to the world. Being something that
never gives in. I have died a thousand times, only
to rise again on the pinions of hope. Hope and the
newness that beckons. I have been told, by
people in the know, that time is a plaything by the
wise and the passionate. We have never seen fate
so strong. And then, holding up from the side, a
foreign clime, a mystery beckons. There is here
something that we have as the gate and the moat.
We will come.

Conscious and awake, we dream of nothing more.
Nothing more of the sand that holds us back, nor
the extremities that are a blessing. Come now,
sounds are here for bleeding, and the greatest
sound is of the sea. And then, like a blanket, we
travel there, and stay the night. We have the
window open. In the morning we head out, and
see what we can see. Pulsing, moving, ebbing,
flowing – everything we could want.

There is now a sense we have that the vastness of the heart is a labyrinth to other worlds. As our heart pounds, we travel to these worlds, and we see ourselves in these worlds – fighting, loving reading, writing. There are dimensions here, dimension to strike accord with. We know that these dimensions are nothing but our dimensions, our world, our adventure – all through the heart. Much is said, much is written. We will find a way.

Vacuous, and in charge. What makes us last. What has the same sound as the breeze on rooftops. What we say to make things better. What we dream of, despite. What is there, and there abouts. What is there for good. Treasuring for the sunlight, as it comes again into our lives. Do you know what it is? It is us, as we standstill and luxuriate. Missing nothing, we often see ourselves here – in difficult times, difficult displays.

Vociferous and multi-lingual. Coming for cover, without the sound of it. Moistening the land. What doesn't fit. I am here to make agreeance – agreeance that can harbour. Not anything else. My levity is the wind. My strength is short. I am the way things are, and the noise that people make. There is entirely one thing, and it is here, like a distance that releases unto itself, and through itself. Fortunate to see, but not what we should come for.

A like-minded degree of relief. A glass that reveals hearts to be sure. What do we say when things are grey? What do we do when the sky hinders rather than harvests? There is a place inside everyone, where, when things are dark, we can come, and settle, and be with who-ever we want – old friends old lovers, old acquaintances – and here, where the imagination is powerful, we can fall into a deep sleep, and simply dream of the limitless possibilities. A place we all have inside, us and the sea.

Disaster, and relief. Two things that hinge on one another. And here, where the sound of angels comes down from the crowd, they know themselves to be the curtailment of absorption. What do the fair and the wounded have in nestled agonies? What does the relief say, that we have not said? I cannot seal the soul of it. There are wings that try and delay, but delay me not. Hold out our hands for the tapestry, it comes in folds.

Fostering gladness. It curtails in satin irregularities. And here, where the dice are not thrown, many things come to the sound of the wishing and the nightingale. Do not hinder us, nothing stops the rock and the forbearance. There is a way forward, and so we take it. Messages are sought, and things that we have achieved are thrown. Do not beleaguer the dame, she haunts for you. Do not carry the satchel, it lingers in the air. Just believe.

Whispering, at night. Falling in the air. A sepulchre in a nowhere land. I come to seek, not to cajole. I come to find love, but where can it be? The heart beats but where is it found? Things are clear, but what of the great message. What do we find when we look? Is this intransigence? Is this the tape that binds us? We look straight ahead, but what do we envisage? A staple in the doorway holds us back. But it is more than that. Things will come, and then, respite.

Chapter 6.

Mingling with reminisces, the time we find does not escape us. And then, a lingering, by the fire and all its worth. We love what we find here. And then – cascade, and the whims of soldiers worn thin. Do not convalesce, such things are written but not embedded.

And now, looking like the stars had wrapped him, there syncopated, with an eruption and an effusion, there like a miscommunication, there like festivities in the train of it. Simply there, like never before. We come off the back of it.

Midnight rituals, and all that can be. Rituals, and the slightest dilemma. Rituals and the mildest pang. We never force ourselves. Only when the time is short, and only in the in-between of times. And now, we come.

There are things in this world that surprise – in many different ways. One is to surprise by stealth. Another is to surprise by way of amelioration. Another is surprise by way of concordance. And others. We shall see what surprises me.

Invective and the will. Invective and the all that is. I have come to play a role – a role to see how far, and how long, and how incumbent. There is now a

play on words that steals itself the right of way.
And here, we must not fall.

Almost capitulated. Close to that thing. But with
help (always with help) we continue. There is
never enough to see. There is an onerous
possibility of the oneiric. Stay in the sense of it, it
will come. But before then – an announcement;
tabula rasa.

Costing what we need to survive. Is there any
price for good health? And then like a solstice that
never wanes, we saunter up to the plains, and
have as our release all the pains of all the world.
There we will rest.

Gesticulating and with a height that shuns all else.
I am one who is walking. I am one who links arms.
I am one who steadies things that are here. And
now, with all the force of all the things, comes a
gathering of ways.

Horsing around, until the light of dark diminishes,
and the wisps of tomorrow begin. There is a light
breeze at our backs, and it carries us forward,
where normally we would take rest. Be the
wounded, and all that we have been through will
come.

Four squared and one. There is nothing to champion causes quite like this. And here, where the mission to save is like a balm, there reaches nothing else in behind. Testing things, we walk a little faster than is normal. We will find.

Much achieved, much in serendipity. Much to be seen, much to be goaded. Much unloaded. Much to see again. What have we thought? What have we given? What is the best of it? See these things, they are yours. Now go find.

I am one to know the price of pain. But I also know the price of difficulty. And in-between the price of austerity. Much is witnessed. Much is thrown. Much to delight, and all to fathom. I will never see the same again.

What do we say, when things are awry? What do we say, when the magnetism diminishes? What do we know, despite all facts? Come now, we must not be shy. What we see before us is a goose ready to fly.

Catching the last of the play, we laugh to see the end. And now, with the sort of feeling that has never transpired before, we move ourselves forward, like rugs on a hessian floor. Do not doubt, the tethers that bind will loosen.

Further from the source than we gather, we motion inward to find our way. It is about the solution of the difficulty. And here, where we are best suited to the cause, nursery rhymes and all things bright. We are here to say

And then, like a feather that does not know the way – invigoration, and the crispness of reality. Find a way through – I hear you say. And so we will – in the fullness of time. And now, the orchard reminds us of things past. We will know.

The sea comes. The heart comes. And when they both combine, there is a sound. All we must do is put our ear to some one's chest when we are by the sea – and that is the sound we hear. Much meaning. Much endeavour. Much learning.

Heaven made thee, but for what purpose? Heaven drained thee...but for what score? Rat-a-tat-tat, fibres in the drift of it. Canning in the sport of it. There is only what is left. There is only here, and now there.

Moisture departs, but what do we really think? What is it that keeps us running, when our legs no longer pump. What is it that we labour with, when labouring diminishes its lot? Come now, chose the way forward, and we will make motions.

Filling quickly, we raise our heads, taller still. And when we come, we do so for the age, and the silence, and the new found relishing. What is lost can be found. What is longed for, will be sent – eventually, and with gusto.

Frosty, and with ice. Never before seen. Lancing with considerable aplomb. Having the figures, and rounding them down. There is enough here to bring glee to the stage. There is enough here to sit for hours.

A lot has happened, and a lot will happen more. But as we go, we see the hill of content move slightly to the left. And here, where we love to be, something of the sand lies down, and says to us – be sound and thoughtful.

And then, like water in a maelstrom, things come to be what they should. And then, like an ambience that steadies us for the show, we never fall behind the line. Come now, mistletoe comes and goes – but hearts do not.

What is more, traipsing through the arena are the Midas men and women that have as their result great tension to sooth and to bind. But what of this? What of this, that we cannot see? We unload our trifles, and see ourselves arch again.

Paul Fearne

What of the sanctity of life breathing life? What can we say of either/or or/either? There is a lot to say, here on the plains. There is much to do as well. But what of the offering of light and sound that treats us so well? In due course.

Mismatch, and heights arranged. Be a token to the kingdom, and yours will be the life. There is now a sense of comradery that sings itself to sleep, and has as its frame the night and all that it contains.

Vestiges, and condolences. Come backs and dissuasions. We have never had more fun than this. And by this, we mean all. Ha – a serendipity of behaviours. We claw back time – but to what effect?

Much in the way of. Much to skirt around. There are times that have no ilk. And reaches that have the sense not to burn. There are things that combine the heart and soul, and then there are things that don't.

A little bit of the harvest to sure things up. Much to be said, on the vine of tomorrow. There is a winding in the trellis. There are coldness's to take part in, and those to keep away from. There will be much time for revelry.

84

We have yet to see the bottom of it. We have yet
to see the heart of it. Closing in with speed, we
never miss a beat. Closing in like soldier's
harshness, we long for the days of it. We long for
the delays of it.

All over this world, there are sounds of remorse.
But what we find when we look, no one has
committed a wrong. Everyone can find
redemption; all they must do is look. And then, like
fire and ice, relief.

And now, with hearts pounding, we start walking –
walking without a destination in mind. It is as if we
could not stop ourselves. And the further we walk,
the further we want to. It just keeps on going,
endlessly, aimlessly.

What is more each step we take, each licence to
breathe, is like a sign in the wind, the wind for all
of us. Never stop giving – it is time to accrue;
accrue the vision filled, and the larrikin. We will
never stop believing in things.

A heartbeat. A sea wave to shore. This is where
we come to the fore. This is where things never
stop. This is where the conundrum is always
resolved. We see things the right way up. And in
these things are those that matter.

Much toil – much to see. There are founding stones that mark no building. There are festivities that mark no occasion. And here, where the moisture comes in unerring waves, there comes a time to settle, take stock, and simply amaze.

Tribulations – for and against. Love in the triangle – for and against. There is little to be said, that hasn't been. And now, with that in tow, we specialise in what comes next. And furthermore, sand in the bucket.

A counter sign, one that rears in times of difficulty, times of hardship. And without a thought, nor semblance of the rest. Be more than the others think is possible. Be more than the wide spread. Just be more, and have-to-it.

A little bit of spice has come to play. A little bit of spice to hold back the day. Wisdom, and compassion. Wisdom and compassion. We have no fear. Nothing can stop us. Give back what was called for. And yours will be all.

A college that gives its all. And despite the changes, we love what ensues. We love it so much, we are tempted to kiln-fire it to make it real. A sense we have that the dates are here to lavish pride upon the group.

Fighting for play, fighting for belief - never one to hold back. This is the time of it. This is the way of it. I hear you say something about the sea? About hearts? About all that is reminiscent. Come for the scaffolding, and then away from it.

Activate the policy. Never to trundle, never very far. Never to be remis, come what may. There is something in the water here, but that cannot stop us. The moisture in the air is phenomenal. Shall we repeat, and then discard?

Having a harrowing time of the wind and all that will pass. I can think of nothing greater than this. There are things we must do, and things that must pass. And here, where the chains that bind are released, we find our circumference.

And now, where the measures of a person are many, I choose not to relinquish fate, and see it flare with so much in sight. I have faith in fate, and know that she is the one that will take me there – so much on the ways of it.

And then, like a belief in the air, solidity and a firsthand glimpse of everything. There lives a long life, much to be partaken of, and much to be believed in. Silence is the key. Silence and the stroke of solidarity. We will see it come.

Let us never remove the counter weight. Let us never remove the weight. We are tall, but our bodily strength is small. We have mental strength, the likes of which is rarely seen. The body follows after.

Coming close to the dust of it, we climb our way higher. Higher into the mass of it. And then, like a bell jar in the midst of it, a sense that charisma can take us there. We will never shirk.

Longing for all the right things. Longing for the stars to collide. Longing for the assets not to fade. And here where the beach is the colour of the sun, the scent we have that time is of the essence. This is what we have.

No more of it – no more of the sound of it. No more of what is tempting us to throw down. There is a way of it to discover. A way of it in the lay of this land. It is majestical, to defy the logic of things. It will come, it has already.

Meshing with grief – a certain sense of calm. And here, where we love to be, nothing stops the challenge, except us. A part that is frozen through. Will we make it, we have to, we will make it to the next station. And then through.

Apart from this, there is nothing that does not collide. Be the way we are, and what you will find, will conquer a nation. I believe in many things – one thing is the sand on a beach directly looking out to sea. Amazing - magnificent.

Sitting directly in the path of life, we then get up and meander through the whistling ponds, and then through the harvest of delight. A suitable stance is found for all. And then, back into play and daggers.

Come now, holding firm – holding back the time, like it was the sea. Holding back what should never be thought. Holding back something special. We will never see these things again. And then what? Agog.

What has come to be, is not so far from the reality. And then, with march hair in hand, we sniff around the corners, and crawl our way there. No one can see us, nobody cares. It is as if we were nothing, but repartee.

I see one thing, and one thing only – the clouds before a thunderstorm. This much I know how to follow. It is as if I weep at the sight, such is my camaraderie. I will have it no other way.

What is left, is not the heart of love, but the love of hearts. What is distant, is not the sea at dawn, but the dawn at sea. Harbour only that which expands your life. And in that motion – see what is best; best and brightest.

Fighting for it. Never letting go. Dispelled, but then returned. A source of disquiet – and then, something truly great. I hear the messenger, and know how to laugh at him. Do not be disturbed – enough.

Fashioning a raft – seeing it through. Being able, and commissioned. There are types of sail that suit. I will not stop until the unleashed beckons – and even then. Wishing for the veil to be completed. We will soar.

The limit of us all, is the limit of us all. Much endeavour, and much to swoop. We linger by the gate, to see what we may become. And here, we taste freedom for the first time. There is no rush – nothing to dispel.

A gladness not to curtail – if we at all can. And then, spatterings of goodwill that sending us flying. And then a rising that buries deep. We have so much to talk about, let us commence – can there ever be an end to this?

A furtive glance is all it took. And then, like a wagon on display at the turmoil, there stands a magnificence that cannot be rivalled. We sit alone, without the need even to do so. And in the mean-time, a gesture of awareness.

Must believe it first. Must have the night and all she is worth. Must be the tempest in a strange and distant land. 'I will use it for my purposes', she says in the dark. A swampy land, that has each troubadour reeling.

A dry and fallow land. A location that doesn't allow reminiscing. Please be the happenstance in a place full of happenstance. Be the wisdom of them all, and yours will be a fruitful surmise.

A ringing true – an allotment that sighs. We have never heard it this way before, but neither have you. Come now, do not be tired, the journey is just commencing. We have many more miles to travel, many more tempests to meet.

Mesmerising, and at loggerheads.
Commiserations, and then, next, and swiftly - all that uplifts. There is a sense we have the things will be okay, no matter what. Things will be okay – no matter what - despite any bedevilment.

A winding up, to let spin – a true beginning, that leaves its mark. We look forward in time, only to see things shine. Only to gather an audible want, something in pieces please, something that harbours the ingenious, and lets fly.

Gosh, and bother. There is a cat on this tin roof – that is fine, we will send ourselves through to be surprised. And then like a new town to be buoyed, a further invigoration to counter the weight.

Let's do it – let us no longer impede progress – let us be not that way inclined. Let the masterstroke be final. Let the dimensions of tutelage run clear. Let all that is going to be fine, be fine.

There is now something that does not condescend. There is now something that scends. And with that, we have said what needs to be said. And that is what tingles on the spine, for one last swing on the chandelier.

Chapter 7.

There is here the stuff of fire-works. And when the time descends, much frivolity, much mirth. Do not dream of anything else. The dreams we have anon sanctify the dreams we once had. And now, without so much as a miserly account of things, the distance we find between this and that place, is like the chestnut and the squirrel. There comes a chance, to defy everything, and in doing so, we stand alone. And stand towards, much that is forgiven.

Much that is timeless, and much that is difficult. Much that knows when, and much that doesn't. I see your work – it harbours on mine. I see your placation – it never denies. There is a sound – it fears, but is founded. It treasures, but like a bridge, draws on. And now I see your space – do you see my space? Is this the harvest and the tithe? I cannot diminish in foibles. There is much to be said of all things. But what of the barley and the cradle?

Trusting things to be, and the belief that they will. What we cloud with our vision, and what we feel can never be let go of. I sense something I haven't sensed since my birth. What is new, is not old. What comes in clumps of clay, is for the road ahead. What we see in our mirrors, is enough blind the way. I sense in tune to mighty incumbencies. Things are good here, we should leave them. There is a turnstile of existence that awaits. Awaits the sighing, and the traipsing.

Crossing the street, we wait till our allotted time. And then, in the distance, a pocket of air – we wait for it, still. And then like a bridge of disinterest, we find the will to cross, and then we are there. A slice of the real comes to us. There is nowhere else to look but here. We find ourself in time to the many and the few. There comes a chance at something greater – and greater still. And that much can we fall for, once that falling is all that we have.

Nestled in strong – little known binaries come to life. I believe, once and for all, the sound of longing is for everyone. Do not say when. Do not weigh in for the travesties of nature. That is for another time. We are set upon by the land we speak of. And here, where the journey meets the sea, much to guide, and much to imbue. I found my way – it is unorthodox as it is steep. It is cautious as it is rounded. We will never know its true scope. We will not bend.

A silent cave, with mounds of what is best. There, there, we are not sleeping. We wander, and walk, and gather ourselves for the road ahead. There is a sound I know of. I have heard it before. It is from a warbling bird. And here, where the pitch of reality rolls the boat, there comes a time for pleasures, and utmost causes. And now, we know exactly what we need to do. Run up that hill. Make that next ridge a milestone. And then what's more, something to hold on to.

A certain way of doing things. A long and crouching approach. What is there now that hasn't been said? What is there now that believes in the future? What have we come to that is not made of time? I hear your call, and echo back with tenderness. What is there to sit upon, that has not the marks of the lion? A corner stone (of sorts) that trails in undue bliss. A ripping yarn, that divvies up a quandary. Never before have we seen something like this.

There is here and now, vast enclosures, that see in themselves the tidings of commensurate by plays, and side plays, and plays that have nothing left to give. There are times we linger – special times. And there are places we go to when life is overbearing. The testament is written in the sky – do not hold back, we see things, but do not run. We are here to see, and here to envisage more than clusters ever could. Forever more. We have that which is whistle determined.

Causing a stir, what more can we do? Things take us, but we take them back, in measures that have not been heard for a millennium. Do not send the gracious to the fickleness of it – it is feared. Instead take a stand, it will fill your being with mirth. I have come to play – play in times of disease. What won't be had, will be the treasures of worn-out pride. This much can be reminiscent of the last. I am bent on calling things by their names, no matter how far we have to go.

Measuring up the litany of remarks we find in the box below the table. There is nothing more to do – nothing more to say. We linger, but for what? We hold hands, but with whom? We come again, but for what purpose? There is mischief in the wind of it. Come now, we are here. Come now, songs are strained. There can only be what we have not forgotten. There is a trace of togetherness here. But what do we do, when the journey slows, and what we have says a solemn – Hey.

Almost at the intersection – where we cannot contain ourselves. There is solemnity here. There is a rage-some feel. There is blistering on the souls of our feet, where the time it takes is not disregarded. There is a plan – a plan we have never seen before. There is a sense that what we see now has been harboured by the tooth and the stone for an age. It comes again, in moisture laden festivals of light. There is now something more that we must invest of ourselves.

Lovingly, and with praise. Never relinquished, but never here. There is like a sport to it. Something we cannot tell in the vision or the cusp of it. We sing, but for what purpose? We love, but for which time? The maelstrom is in the head – but how do

we find it? There is a catacomb of desire here –
something truly belated. But do not be for it, it
comes in gradients of life. The job we do here, is
like a summer's day – bright, but too hot. Do not
be attuned to one so attuned.

In the distance a newly won composure.
Something we have longed for, but now have. In
this box, a rounded gem casts its light through
world in equal measure. There is no way to tell
how far, or how strong. There is only the motion of
light to guide us. And then, like a catapult over the
tower – things believe once again. This much is
clear – so clear. But what is left, is never close
enough. There is now a tale to tell – and we shall
tell it – not before too long at least.

A drudge to go there – but to see! There are
passages of time that have as their mast all the
reckoning of the while. Massage the clock until it
turns full circle. Come what may, we hear the way
things go. And then, a portal to see through, one
last time. We do not see our lot, only that we are
there. Do not sport the treasure of it – it seeks
itself in grey, in modes of white. There is now
something vision filled, as much as can be
expected. We will find the lever.

 Grasping for air, we see ourselves not moving in
a sea of doubt. What we must do is to swim
against the tide, in a way remarkable for its
veracity. There is no time to transcend the mists of
dilapidated inquiry, all we can do is look past the

time, and then see things once again in light of a different shade. And then, like the proverbial, we spin on acres, and have what is left of the shadow's march. Come now, do not be concerned, shadow's language is cool to the touch.

Withering, but sewing, sewing the seeds of ardour. There is a likeminded harvest to come, so be plentiful in time for the wastrel's land. There is now nothing like the mist to come in a benchmark of beauty. See the Hellespont revoke its name. See what comes next disregard all but the trappings. See what comes next haul in long vein. Be the simplicity of it all, and your reward will be endless. Do not come up short, the road here is potholed. Believe in one thing – the intrepid.

Art, and the makeshift – hearing on boards of grey. There are soundings, in this way and the next. Soundings that have as their pleasure all the tenacity of the wolf and the squire. No longer will we saddle our horse after watering. No longer should the time take us there. We must entreat the layers to all that we hold dear. And then, like a fish in the deepest blue, congratulations, you have made your companion new. What have we thought otherwise – never.

What is at liberty, is not the sea – not the heart – but two conjoined things that gel as one. There is never a space to speculate equations, or find the round where the two of them lay. What is more, forgetting dimensions for a moment, laughing is the way of all things. We nestle in quarters made from silk, and are harassed no less from the deep of it. Come to the season, have fall, the way of all things. There is a message from one thing to the next – it says, 'yes, movement, yes'.

A distance – what does it matter? Nothing if you will it. See the same again on the rooftops as we bridle a new passion. Just in time to see what comes next. There is a line in the wilderness, that has as its rasping, the furrowed brows of the few, and the dreamt to be quarters of the aspiring and the clasping. We come this way only in the middle of things. A fruition of particles, they transpire, as we call on life to be our resumption. Never once, always twice.

What is the heart, but the sea. Our human imagination contains this space, so our claim is not too heady. The whispers of glee fork out, and have what we need. There is a stunning reception we receive from the stone of it – stunning in completion and in vision. Be the broth – hope will stand still. There is a champion in the guard. A champion that rules in ascendance. What do we make of this now, we call for more – and with more venom and more bite.

There is a task at hand, one that sees the natural jeopardy in reigns of silk, reigns of disarray. The meaning behind the saying is found in the start of things, a place that we all find in the maelstrom. Live large – there is nothing else to it. Live for the time it takes. Live for the fizz of it. There is really nothing else too it. I take your hand, and know that things will be fine. Take my hand, and see what may come, and overcome it instantaneously. That will be seen as a tribute.

Forests containing the fruit of release. Forests containing all that is. There is nothing more in this – forests live for us. And wait for us as does the dawn. Which comes first – the forest or the dawn? It is not is not rendered through any known shape or form. Be the soul of it, heart will come. Be the likelihood of tears, and measurements will not become you. Considerable need we have. Considerable approaches we will have. One thing stands out, love and its embrace.

A vast encounter that cries out into its own. There is something here. What is it? It knows only too well that the floor is made for crashing, and the laughter of the Czars is here. We hear our own laughter, and simply know. We simply know all that we must. Come and see what we have in turn. Have in turn in the daylight, and all that reckons by her. There is something here – something we have not seen before. This much will keep us going.

A sycamore tree, that has as it feeling all the world. We see now why it has come, why it is here, and what it will become. There is now something auspicious, something intriguing what's more. We never relinquish the time. Not today at least. Not today, and also not tomorrow. We chain ourselves to the need of it – to sense of it. There is something in the way of the dance. Something moves with wonderment. We will find a place to be still.

Measuring a stick – to be thrown at the wind. A concerted effort not to be outside. There are places that have no want, and gurgling that has no respite. Divide the plateau, with every solemn breath. Divide that which has no heart. The sea then stays whole. There is a chance in amongst it to see the flowers bloom - a magical thing. Ride the tremendous motion of a ceiling full of life. Can you see the patterns? They are surely there.

A magic that we are yet to see here. A magic that buries in deep. We are forsworn to always renew. We are tempted to always leap at things – leap at things in the dark. That makes us treasure what we have. All we have, and then some. What is it now? What can we see without? Magisterial, and all that comes to pass. What of it? What of it now? We may cease upon any recommendation. But the tide – does it hear? Does it face itself in dead of night? Only motion can tell. And only then without us.

And now with hindsight engaged, we lurch forward to the roof of our souls. It is here that conundrums cease, and foreboding likewise. There is great release, and auspicious returns – but what of the delay? What of the sound of it? How far does it travel? We may never come back. That much is true. A verging, and a placating. Never once have we seen this. And now, a stranger appears. He is handsome, and diligent and knows our names. He will help.

Menacing at first, and then slowly calming. What is this thing we call respite? What is this thing we need upon resumption? A lot of help, say all and sundry. Give the rainbow its due – it to can help. We see its beauty in silence – there is nothing like it. And then, as a sense of pride emerges, new found longing, and everything that is in due course. I will find a way to be in times of difficulty. And here, what we know to be a relic, is nothing other lines drawn in the sand.

And what now? What of the vestige? What of all the things in-between. Do they rinse, and then move on – on to prior grounds. Sounds likewise. An addition to the status quo. A foundling disrupts, and then like a noise in the distance, something else comes – what is it? First in tethers, an unlikely passage. Second in the guise of it. Thirdly with heart, straight from the sea. We gather, and know the worth of things. Touchstone, and the newness of it. We pin our hopes.

Fossils, and reputations amongst it. We sit keenly forward, and know that in a moment, things can change. There is here the willing of an age, in-between heart-beats, and part-beats, and all that beats. Sounds too, let us not forget them. All we need is a likeminded approach to render this life acceptable. Do not contend with the unruly, theirs is a life of mystery, and sense and charm. All the more ready, as time goes by. All the more in score.

Fortune, and the bracing of iron wings. There is here something we must not watch. Something that has as its base more than we could possibly imagine. More than hearts can feel, more than cherished deliveries. More than is like the wind, and all that she can dispel. I have felt my shape, around trees of wisdom's folly. I have felt the wind around the trees, and up and back again. The noise of patch work follows us to the touch.

Witching the way through, we find ourselves with tougher souls and tougher heart-beats. And then, like a harvest that enjoys its own delights, something appetising we find on the journey through. Motion that installs all the rain in the world. We have left here the scars of another nomenclature. What we have is between you and me, and all the stars in the sky. Veritable and ensconced. Veritable and enamoured. What is more, is having two hands to fit it.

Converging on windswept hills, there is a great abandon we have only recently recognised. And here where souls sleep in time to marching orders, a left placating signature hands over the mass. What we have found, is that the sound of sycamores does only enough in the right places. And this means rest for us. And rest for you. I leave you a card to get by. I sense in this more than the wrangling of fireflies in dead of night. There will be a reluctance.

Like the wary, and the little. Like the might, and the consolidation. But the consolidation of what? Dreams and all that undulates in the valley. All that finds itself alone in this oblique world. Do we catch the rise of it, such that the marks of tension are relieved. Is this what we find when we look? Is this what we have when we find? Much to be envisioned. Much to race for the accord. Much encased in sand. Much imbued by the storm – we will never encounter more.

There is a crying in this place. A crying that never seems to leave. But what is left, when it goes, is nothing short of perfection. And here, where the misanthrope resides, much mirth as well, and much laughter and much to gather. There are things we must not abide, and things we must. But here, despite ourselves, we give money to the wise, and see gestures unreal to the normal touch. There are windings down corridors of ancient buildings that no longer feel the way. But despite, we have it.

In time to life, there loves a novel way of being, one that doesn't see itself as anything other than riches and boredom. And here, where the time of it flees the floor, much to sense away with, and much to do battle with. I cannot see the chance in this that heralds more of the concave, and less of the convex. What do we do when this is the last thing we do? We laugh, and play and besiege the space in between this theatrical show and the next.

There is now a temperance that holds in sway more than the forest floor – more than the windswept desert – more than the raging sea. And it is here, we realise ourselves as people to learn and respect, respect others. But what of the mystery of it – that which comes to be in time with most things. Half-way there, and still relishing the night. Diminishing there, and always on guard. Acclimatising here, and nothing we can do to stop.

There is light in this antechamber – light through and through. There is something more to, something we at first failed to understand, but then picked up, and ran with it. And it is here where we finally made the connection. It is here, that we knew ourselves for the first time. It is here that time remained still. It is here where we first made motions. There is nothing sweeter in the mind than that which encompasses. We will see more of the dawn.

Misting with the hallmarks of life – we return from leagues below. We never have been deeper. But what we missed is not the air above (although that was a factor), but the depth deeper below. We couldn't go any deeper. But what we say to the wind, now that we are back, is something of the sort of – chase my back, I am here to stay. There is never anything we could do than is greater than this. The sea is solemn my friends – let us dance.

Ascribing tenacity on the wall of hardship. What we thought was that we could write our way through it – and that we did. Much to see in this life. Much to dream of. Much to settle. I will come full circle before this is arranged. What can we say, that has not already been said. What of the window that looks out onto the sea? What of the stones in the garden that never move – shall we try and move them? There is only one answer we can give – yes.

A type of quiet – that acquires itself new found longing. What does not diminish is the sound of you and me and we talk about the weather, and see ourselves in new garb, something to show off to the neighbours. There is a sort of plaintive approach, that has as its direction the might and solace of an empire in waiting. Considering this, something we have not issued, is the breeze as it blows in a diagonal motion. We will follow where it goes.

Come and see this. Come and see the turn of things in much considered, new light. There is a having to tread, and there is a wishing to be said. We are at liberty to sample on one cloud at a time before we are away. Lost and in method, we catch the distance with an ochre embrace. Here is now a silence in the wings. Let us hear it for a brief time. And get ready, to hear something special from nature. There we are. It will hold

There is something more pronounced, than what is left in store. Come, and be what is true, until the sky spills red. Be a match stick to the dawn, and set the world on fire. We must never remain in stasis. We must never remain in love. And it is here, where the embrace lasts the longest – it is here that sounds of laughter, sounds of tears mark our canvas. How else do we express this? How else do the horizon and life converge? We will never know.

Caution here, there is a breeze afoot. Cautionary and needful of the thread bare. Customary, and changing all the time. Is that what has got us here? Change and bareness of willow. I will have nothing of it. There is a time for play, and a time for work, and a time to listen, and one to envision. It is as if the ground had fallen away, and ankles were needed to balance. Be the tempest it will not hurt, not hurt one bit. Watch for the candles, they hold more than we can tell.

Vagabond whispering, vagabond hailing, wishing for things ashore. Wishing for the tail lights. Wishing for what is left. There comes a cross roads reeling, a cross roads harkening. What is here, is not there. What is there is not here. What we gather has the craft to it. What we gather has a sense to it. What is more, it feels the way. What is sempiternal feels the same. There is like something we have never experienced. There is a way forward, and it marks the in-between.

What is this that we find amongst the fibres? What is this we search for, day and night? What do we clamber for, inside and out? What does only diminish us in halves? There is a well-spring that we know not of its source. There is a listing on the seas of fate. There is something to do, and something not to do. A little piece of fumbling in the dark. What we curtail so it does not hurt us. What the regions of the heart speak of. Come now, do not splinter.

What is left of our ease? What determines the path to come? What elevates us, and then is there afterwards? A dream of something forthcoming. A situation of the betrothed. A wondering that holds hands. Is this where we stand – on shallow legs? Do not scurry, life has us both. And believe you me there is nothing to do but follow. The sea is of the heart. This much we see. But the heart is also of the sea. Conjoined in unison.

Night-time – Night-time and the strange. Night-time and the story of us. Night-time and all that can be. What we sense is nothing other than well-being as she harbours the mist, and tuns with it. Can we feel the solstice? Feel the solstice in graduated light? There is a pound of snow ready to embark. Not here, but there. Not there, but everywhere else. Come now for the show of it. Come now for the test of arms. We will know when to balloon in pleasure.

Chapter 8.

Clawing at the delicacy of it all. Fusions of light
and sound. There is not a moment like this –
anywhere. We know what we are told. We know
what we should do. But here – here, there is a line
in the sand. And it is here (oh here) that we fetch
the dust off the mantle piece. And in this way, we
do not settle – we do not for anything.

Much trouble, to get it right. But here, where the
Fjord lies temperate, a much-heralded synopsis,
going to the middle, and then beyond. We see
ourself in joy, and in splendour. What is this, I hear
you say? Convalescing – convalescing from life.

Fortune, and waste – terms for another era. What
more do we need, than particles of window rain?
What do we say then, than other and over? There
is now transport inclined to be – and so will us, in
the shape of it.

Spoiling and the rushing. There are times to sit
and learn, and then there are times we fly like
magic. And then in-between something else –
something that cannot have a label attached.
What is this – something quite exquisite.

Nobody and the highest harness. Nobody, and the
further we have come. There travels more of the

future than of the past. But what of the now? We see – it is in the frame. Much harmony, and much to do. We will work.

Causing a ruckus, but then, calling out a name, and hearing your name returned. This is the way in should be. This is the way it could be. Forever tender, and then forgiven. There is much to be said.

Cascading down and through. Glimpsing all we can. And here, where reason turns to passion, gains turn to sweat. We launch forward in a movement that does not stop. And here, where the mission to betroth launches from one place to the next, I see myself caught in the crossfire, and know all to be fine. And more.

A certain type of fire, one that never breathes. One that contains the sundries, and all the quiet of the marsh. I have as the letter, latter-day incumbents. And now, forward thinking, as we stretch for a rest. Come and be seen, there is no means to it.

A depth that has no bottom. A top that is free with no limit. We catch ourselves without thinking. We catch ourselves before the precipice, and then, relax. Things are near, and things are far, and what we find can never retreat.

Forests that have the lives of everyone. Forests that have the needs of the free. We catch a hold of something short of everything, and know that life is here for the taking. We gather, for one last occasion.

Foremost in our minds. Foremost in our hearts. Foremost, and it is time. Reaching for the tendrils, reaching for the past. Reaching for the tethering, that leaves us reeling. Come for this, and be one with things.

A magic that holds sway. A certain type of feeling, that we once knew, and know remember well. There comes a science to it. There comes much of the motion towards it. What is this we see? Silence.

Much like before, hurdles to come, hurdles to jump. We see them, and know our legs to be steady. There is a height to them, that knows one thing – over. And that is like the call of the wild – we will find a way.

What we thought was nothing, has turned into something. And this something, in the end, falls short of anything to worry about. There is a plan to see through what it means to be, and what it means to say.

There is time ahead – time to be fulfilled. And then, like a banshee in tight spaces, we see ourselves approach, and know that we will banish the dark, unto light arcs, unto the day. There can be nothing else.

Continuing on in threes, the trees we see burst together, from the forest, from all else. What have we got, that doesn't blow, or doesn't saddle? The middle of this is something we have yet to pin down. We will come.

There is nothing short of the perpendicular to worry about. And here, where the sand lies diagonally, something we fight for every day. And now amended coursings that trigger new memories, memories of the old.

Falling ahead, in spits and spurts, there is a train of equal proportions. Do not see the feather for the chime of it. Do not believe in the tussles of might, they only disregard the past, and attempt to conquer the future.

Forward, and forthwith. There is much to be said. And here, where the silver of the stone magnifies our appreciation, much sweet sorrow remains. And much that can be tamed, outright. We will never suppose again.

A fire within – a fire without. A fire without water. We cannot see ourselves for the blurring – but strong outline is the key. There is here enough to trade a nave for a princess. But will this do? We shall see.

Posing for delight, there is nothing to it. Posing for the rest of it – it will come. I know of no other form of temperance – just keep going. There is space amongst the debris, kingfishers amongst the rocks – do not dream of respite – it will be here.

And now, without the kind of surprise that can carry a load – I will find the once off distraught, and give the fibre of life. There is nothing left of the sky, the sky, and that which says bye. Much time is spent – it will be.

A falconer, and the breeze at our backs. We know of consideration beyond our station. And now, like a concourse for the gods, something that never lingers, something that hurls itself through and amongst.

And like a renegade troop, we sense the need to wander – to walk the mile as we see it – the mile as we know it to be. There is grass through the hills, and sense amongst the valleys. Nothing is more like this.

A certain magnetism that shines. A certain magnetism that binds. A certain magnetism that does not unwind. There is a belief in wonder as something that can untie the knots of first oblivion. And then? Much.

There are places left untouched by life. And here, where the quantifiable knows how it must comport itself – a semblance to the stars, and all that glitters – We will know the vestige from the source – and that will be enough.

A cascading that covers us in water, and here, in sand as well. This much we know – that in the well-spring, corners that migrate will never submit – And here where value means being decisive – A new course to accrue.

In magic, and in sport of – A cheshire in the night – I am the one to see things anew, and in flight – come to my sanctuary – I hope you endeavour – There is a likeness to the dawn – I see the sea – I hear the heart – let us depart.

In the mode of – In the treasure of – in all insouciant mannerisms, we will come – we will bristle, and leave in water. Come to this tribe – there is a motion – a motion to stop all things. There we have it – impressed?

A lot like the moisture in the air – it comes in strides that have no mission, and further guide to rapturous applause. Be the testimony for the souls of all-clouds – and then, with greater charge, we fight – fight the fight of longing.

Not tethered to the crowd – not unleashed upon the morrow – We see ourselves as a moon in shining light – In dimensions of what are good and right – I will not have stasis, only in the spring. There is hope, and height.

A nonchalant approach that never wavers. A window that breathes – what is more, noise in times of difficulty. Is this what it is? To follow fate and allow not tenderness. There is a rushing here – a rushing in true light.

A fashioning and a caring, not known to any person, or anything. Niceties that see clearly, and fetch nothing robust – we hear ourselves inclined to fabric – fabric that does not diminish. There will be time.

An insistence we have to wade in time to the beat of the sea – This is where we flourish – this is where we are glad to have hearts that pulse. What is more, there shines a talon, the sort of thing we need.

A kind of simplicity that leaves nothing behind (nor ahead). What drives it forward? What has it as a curse? What never lingers – nor gives recompense. What is the system here, that has no domain? We will languish.

And now, with heart and soul in steep alignment, we give the growing esplanade a good look. And then, despite the treasure we find, we look over our shoulder for one last time. It is here – it is here.

A lot like the mission to hang our head, and then have it raised, in simplest motion. Do not deliver the wind unto the foreshore – it will surely come. Do not heather the shoulder of it, it comes to play a foreign role.

A lot like the rest, we do not see ourselves, only others. And then like a bull in winter we catch ourselves panting, and then prancing, and then going forward, not backwards. This is what it is like.

An alignment, one that never rejigs. What the smallest part reminds us of. What we distance ourselves from, but at the same time stay close to. Is there a playacting? – I hope not. And then a tense in quarters – happenstance.

We come close to things anew, and then give a ruffian a throw. Here where silence is prized – we never know what the doorway says. Ambitious, and with halting distance, we call once again for the shore. In this we are sure.

A museum of the everyday. For each person represented, something different. And then like moulds in sky, dancing. The museum holds true to all. There is never a missing dimension here – we must continue.

Targeted from the shore, we know which way to go. And here, the single thought we have is simple – Never for one single moment hesitate. That much is palpable – that much is assured. And then, like a wish in darkest straits, we let go, and swing.

A first-rate swab – for the healing of wounds untold. There is a place for the medical adjuncts, they are quite superb. And here, like elsewhere, we fight the need we have to settle, and find again the fight inside.

Sought for, and loved – never once believing in things that digress. What is the way through here? What do we seek, when seeking is of the age. A commission, to consign the largo to outer flanks. This much can accrue.

Safety, and inner freedom. Enslavement, and tailoring of invigoration – there comes a liberty, that doesn't need the touchstone nor the hearse. There are now things unrivalled – and indeed unplanned. Let us go – let us depart.

What we need, is what we find. What we find, is what we need. Countenances massing on the streets, never once believing in hopelessness. A sense that things will become right again – Never once denying.

Listening closely, having quite the time of it. There is a way forward. But how? Simple – all we do is turn our wings skyward, and launch. That is one way at least. The others are here to drive – watch them, they will come.

Recourse to wonder, and to the stellar. Recourse to winter and that which can only fly. Do not recant on the journey, it knows you. It is hard now, and cannot be harder. But when things have settled, they will fall into place.

Much in the way of love. Much in the way of sustenance. Much not too obscure. There is a kindness here. That transcends all else. What do we want from it – what do we dare. There are figures in the mesh of it – look and see.

There can only be the night, so have a notion that walks, walks and says right, we are fire, fire to abandon. Have something else to say – nothing too quick, or too slow. Nothing on the baggage of it – that is the rule.

Fetching the congress of it – we travel in shards of the spectacle. And then, without a sentence to utter, we mistake our eyes for blindness and still, despite, travel to where we want to go. That will be enough of it.

There is something magical here. I don't know how, or why I say that, but I do. There is so much at odds with personal happiness, but we can't ridicule life, it just is. And then with a startle, we begin.

Considerable pleasure, that is languid in form, and despite its customary appraisal, gives respite to those who journey. I feel my way to the epitome, and give way to the sense of it all.

And then, with gushing pride, the spheres move again, in circular embodiment. The nearest treatment does not suffice in time nor accolades. There is a thought that if the world stood still, mirrors would cease to work.

Gravitating towards an accustomed solace, there is here, life to be had. What sort of life, we do not know – but life is life. There is a magnitude to be given, and sought after, but that is in time to the most indignant of us.

Galvanise – a special word. There are somethings we go through to do just that. A vibrancy – the treasure of any word. What delivers, is not the sound of it, nor the wind – it is the concourse which appears – we love it.

Vindictive, and soluble. Intransigent and insatiable. What we have, but do not have. What we sight at a distance, but do not love. A meadow that cries out – we will come. There is danger in the eves – we will relinquish.

Forthright and forthwith. A special symposium of the heart. We place our heads side on and press against the chest. A recording of the sea at high tide rings out. There is more here than we can possibly imagine.

Fetching the sand at a whim. What do we find but a certain noise, sounding like a sea-shell lapping up water. There is here licence to do as we will – but we refrain ourselves, just that one more time at least.

There is a clasp, she once wore, I have looked everywhere. When I find it, I will give it back to her. But for now, I search – search for what? Search for the centre, the centre of a worn out being – she was my centre.

A kite in the sky. Two-fold high. We will never forget this moment. It is like we have won at everything. Keep the linoleum for yourself. There is now a fortune hunt. One that settles as it breathes.

This section of the library is simply for stars and satellites. Won't you come with us, and tell your story? Is this what it means to grow, and set your sights that little higher? Do not come down, that is your lot.

Where there was dilapidation, there is now the thrill of it. Where there was once a cry in the night, there is now a host of things. I have not heard, in one hundred years, about a time like this. We will find a way.

And then, like a thunder from above, new seasons to rival the old – new fashions to climb up the ease of adventure, and longings that can't seem to be replaced. There – that is now said.

There is a fairytale that has as its chair, a piece of carved wood. On the top of this wood is a book. In this book are some words. And these words are used to inspire people to overcome what they want to overcome.

And then, like a mist we are chained to, a novice at heart comes, and sees the world afresh. There is a task, one that does not labour, and one that does not sing. There is here priceless abandon. Let us through.

What is more, the tethers that bind us have no recourse to sound nor sight – they are easily escaped from. And then, like a motion before dawn, we are swept before ourselves, through a castle, into a moat. And then – yes, then.

Hopeful of the charm and the whereabouts, there is now a sense that the timing is all we need. There comes a great sigh – one of relief. There comes a great feeling – one of sentiment. And this we applaud – for now.

We love with heart. We dance with soul. We have what is needed most. And then, like a labyrinth in the sky, a touch of the simplicity of things. You must know the way here – the way you are walking. Yes.

Chapter 9.

Commencing, but not leaving yet. A hollow on
board, that gives from necessity like the rest of us.
And then, like a gliding mass, we shed a small
number of tears. But what are these? What do we
fence past that is not worth the doing? What do
we see through, that has not a single thing to hoe?
There is now a simple thing to ask. And that is to
rise up, and do the things we have always wanted.
See the renovation of the ages. It will leave you
uncluttered in your own life.

Gleaning – but for what purpose? Concentrating,
but for what reason? There is a time and place for
these sorts of things, and we will take them. There
is a listening that defies all invectives. There is a
plane to remember, across and up. And then like
seashells on the banks of the Nile, we see all our
derivatives lurch and them fumble. This is one we
can definitely see approach. And then, despite all
pleasures, we ourselves fumble – but then catch
ourselves – anon.

Having something more to say, like rocks on the
canvas, like tweed in a dress, like the fibres of this
being, built not to fray. And then, without much
time left, to swing from everything. I have a
raising, that seems neither here nor there, neither
one nor the other. But in reality, it sustains me,
and lets me breathe, and lets me know, that life is
real, and that I am real. But when things quieten,

here, then things become clearer. And we see ourselves together in gold thread.

I am fitted out in sea-spray – that much I know. I also know, that my heart beats for a world on fire. But what of the alias of these things? What of the cannon of all repute? There is now a thing to say – and that is, a gracious 'Hello'. And then like silver in the wind, a traipsing around, or above - 'Despite the handcrafted, we know of no other place like this' – 'Thank you, I would invite you in but we are cold. Come anyway, we treasure all visitors.'

Grainy, and at one with the daylight. Never forced, only cajoled. A strength in nature – we will emulate. Come and envision things clearly. What we have seen at the edge of things, will suffice. There is something that we cannot readily attach to. And that is the time of it all. We will our way to the river, only to find the rains have made it rage. So we must wait, and that we do. There is a moss here we have not seen the likes of. We will make it.

Witchcraft, and sensibility. Openness, and the wrong way to go. There is a passion in square one, that believes itself to be the corner of our eyes. Do be the finish, when the finish overcomes. And with brevity, the target we sight has as the split, a way forward amongst us. There is a type of feeling, that utmost relies on tigers in nightly regalia. And then with a sort of height, we guide the ship, and have it move from waters of residual, to the waters of nigh faring.

A missive in tangential light. There is something more we must be aware of – the tune we seek is not at odds with the parsimony of it all. Not at odds with the template and the canal. We know one thing – there is now a harvest in times gone past. There is now a tempest in times to come. And then with luck hard pressed, a science of it all comes to the fore. What is this science? It is a method of furthest compartments, and the furthering of a still longing.

Containing all – all that will be. Containing all the whims of all the people. Containing all that cannot be, containing the treasure of the long gone. Containing the sense we had to let it be. There is a sound – and in this sound, is a touchstone. And in that touchstone is a vibrancy. And here we know we have the strength we need to pass all tests, and then be the thing that willows in brightest gale. There is more to it than that – our flesh will show the marks.

Much like the last time – we have come to tell a story. We have come to tell the story of life and love, of belief, and of strength. What draws us all together. What keeps us all apart. What is nestled here, but the lounge and the obstacle. We have no time for obstacles, but let us throw the handle into sand. There is a motion that never ceases. There is a landfall that counters all. And then like a dredge, we come up for air, and know it to be sweet. There is time.

Much encumbered – much incensed. We never know what is here, until the dimensions unfold. A crochet of delights are here. And then, like mannerisms on hold, we catch our breath for one more day, and know that time can never really standstill. There is a lark that we can never see. A lark that carries banners of the neverness through wind and rain and steaming moss. There is a likelihood that the moisture hangs perpendicular. Come and see.

Messing around, we come to something serious and that is where we should stop. But as is usual we continue on, and what results is a ramshackle hut in the type of no-mans. There is a taste of it written on the wall at entry. And then, from the middle of nowhere, a bright light which passes as quickly as it has come. We look around, hearts pounding, and we see the centre of it. There is a large space at the rear, with two chairs. We will find a way. Yes we will.

Match box city. There is nothing to see, and nothing to do. But we find something. And in the air above, we see with clarity, and with love, and with compassion. Lots now holds us, and lots to envision. The sense we have that light is here for the taming, is something we cannot shake, nor be relieved of, however far we travel. Can we see ourselves for the new? Can we see ourselves for what is tethered? First we must be untethered ourselves.

Our sight is your sight. Our dress, is yours. Our laughter, your laughter, our sense your sense. There is something more here, than we can see. There is something that never really lets go. But that is okay – but how do we find it? How do we see it? There is here an adventure waiting, why not try to find its source – like the source of a river, a river never coming to rest. What is this, I hear you say? We will come in full swing, and never step down.

Much building, and much persuasion. Much in-between times, and much to let fly. There is now a lot to think about, when the distance only matters twice. Furrowed and without favour. A new type of wrangling, one that wrangles the heart. What more is left of sea? Even if the sea disappears it will still have a sound. Even if there are no humans left, we will still hear their hearts beating. There is a symmetry in this – one that will always be known.

Magisterial and divine. Love and all that passes. We will win this game you and I. And here, where the most is played in twos, there resides a mismatch of rivals. It is here where the battle lines are etched in metal. It is the battle of souls we speak of here. Lives lost, and beliefs tendered, and the journey of the tempest commences. There is heart here as well as being. Thirst, and the wonderment of existence. We plan, two ways to go – up and down.

There is here a sort of wash – one that comes from the sea, and levies itself unto new ways, and past ways. The thing we hear the most is that we cannot abide the ringtail nor the bat. There is here a mischief of sizes. But without much left to do, let us find the puzzlement we cling to, and release the undulating charm. And here where the noise of tomorrow rings true, there casts a pre-eminent assault on beliefs untendered. Here we sit then, above it all.

A like-minded foreboding, much in the trance of fate, much we see in the tower of plenitude, there is the windswept, and gold to be set. Do not be trumpeted by the wind – it is a farce – one to be avoided. We cast aside our lot, and then take it back. There can only be one outcome – and that is to be brief before leisure A residue of relief burns the stage. A reluctance to hear again. But what is here? What is it that stays? Nothing.

We dream – but of what? We are submerged, but by whom? There are questions here, but who writes the answers? Do we come before, and seek a shelter? Is this our lot? To fade in sequence of all that is? We love, and blast the tune above and below. There is like something we have never seen before. Do we let it stay or do succumb to the barbs of tempest squire? There is enough said of this for now, we will wait.

A link in another's chain, we sally forth, and know the distance to be true. Be loath to state indifference, and the time cannot be closer. We follow passion, and passion only – and then, like a well-spring in noon-tide, a love of laughter, and all the rest – we dance – we dance the dance of resilience. We dance, until the screen is divergent. There is now life. We see it, until we can see no more. We feel it – until we can feel no more

Watching, absconding, knowing when its time. There are ways to see things, and ways not. I am of the belief that things come in threes. No three, no event. And here, where the night sheds its garb so festively, there is like a catacomb of wincing, that lights up the street. We have found what we have been looking for. And here, like gold, we retrace our footsteps to ancient places, and all out forgiveness. There is a place for all of this – do not be concerned.

A falconer sees the way forward – they have a habit of doing that. And then with likes of all included, there is a method to these wings, that beat so heavily in the air. And now, like a ragging rock pool we gather ourselves for one more dream. Do not just be satisfied with this – embellish yourself with wonders. There is time here to harvest like never before. Time never to relinquish. Never to translate that fire and the ice. Be that as it may, we will come like never before.

Several sandwiches cannot block our way. And the path is now clear. We hold ourselves with due respect, and know that each passing kiss delights as it diminishes. There is a hidden trap door, that barks out loud. And here, where noises never sing, we hear the sound of a hand in the wind. And it is here, here where we laugh in key – in key to what? – To the world, the sea, the heart, all that passes for reticence.

Mostly enthralled – mostly ensnared – mostly spouting reluctance, on the brim. There is here sense to guide us, and carry us away. Do not feel ourselves ranging through, there is here the most of people lounging, of people crying out, of people seeing things squarely. Not now do we see things in the way of it. There comes a way to be, and much a way to be free. The light in here is ghastly, we will never recover.

Breaking through, scorching the liberty of it. And then, like ten knives hidden, a great escape. I see you tied – tied to the stake, and then like coffee at three in the morning, a motivation that is unstoppable – something that tends itself to the rainbow, and then off again to where ever. There is something in the way of it – what is it? What is this thing – ah there it is, right here. I come to you again, oh might of might. Do not believe there is something. Come for forgiveness, and it will settle.

Open for all hours, we bend once again on the tightrope There is now something that we have not forgotten, for any piece of land on any ground. What is that you have just said? Can we come to the party after six? The boisterous and listless. We have a heart, we hear the sea, and that much can be said. I know of no other wrangling more entrenched. Come then, what is this thing we seek? What is this great thing we speak after? It will rain.

A third of what we normally have them for. Your dreams. Your way of rejoicing, your needs, your delivered speeches – your incumbency, vast as we know it is. And then there is this – the need you have to converse – all for a third off. We rejoice, at things not lost, we have as a heartache more of this than is purely possible. And then like a nightfall we always remember, we come full circle, and then even around again. What is this I tell you? More than we can say.

We watch, and know ourselves to be secure. What does this mean? It means all. What does it say? It says all. What do we know of? Everything – what is there space to say? Like the sense we have that everything will be fine. Like water in the well. Like a clear spell of rain – like all this, and more. I need you to tell me something. What is this dirge we hear? What can be done about it? And which side of the lake is it on? There can be no difference.

What are we fighting for? What is this that holds us? What do we scrape through for? Are our knees bloodied, our palms (slightly)? There is something at ease with this painting. It is of the sea – it is of the heart. The heart is in the sea. The sea is rough, and not abated. The heart beats with the rhythm of the sea. What more can we say? What more do we allow ourselves to be? There is room here for any known regret. We will find our sea legs and go from there.

Further kindness – do we excuse the vice-royal arrogance, for the thing we find in the darkest of recesses? This is what we have fought for. This is what the time has said will come. A nice way, this way, if you enjoy the topsy turvy, and the way to speak. Come now, destinations are ardent, but the gulf between is covered in snow. You must always trust yourself – and in this is a truth – to trust yourself is to never let go. In all the blight of earth, we rise above.

A fork in the road. Even, cross-roads. Which way do we choose? Which way to go? A piece of knowledge – if you hesitate too long, you go nowhere at all. Simply choose a direction, and follow it with your heart, and you have the destination you want. Choose and go. And then, like in a puff of smoke, the magician appears in a different place – you are that magician, and you can follow that puff of smoke wherever we want to go. Do not feel remote, things will come.

Then there is the upside. And that is cherish where you live, and find time for whatever you want. Find time for these things, and your heart will be full. Find time for these things, and what will come will not be a burden. What will come will not concur with any pain nor any evil. There is a foraging beyond life, that has as its fortune the very strength of what drags us on. And what is this – our memories of the sea, and the sound of each of our hearts.

There is now a joy in living through. Living through what may come, and what may be. But what is this? We search deep down, and in that search, we find something, something we can latch onto, and then very casually we look to see what it is, and to see if we can use it. It is, as if, we are sailors in our own water, and here, if this is what we are, it is here, where the marrow of our adventure becomes apparent, and we can see once again.

Blissful, if not a little uncomfortable. And then, like blades of grass – we tiptoe through, and know with a knowledge, of where it comes from, we do not comprehend. There is further we can go here. There is a linkage that knows no chain. There is a chain that knows no destiny. Furthermore, silence begets the scene, which witticism has as a tumult. There is no delay, only a sway, from this side to that.

Marshalling so much, we congregate in the middle of it all. But what is that left here, when the doors are left open? There is here, something to be said, and then like a fibre in the making of it, a silence that has no boundaries. Which do we come for, the silence or the said? There is a making of something special here – something that can only be reproduced in the flow. And then like a marble in the terrarium, we come crashing in. This will do – and do nicely.

And then, like rock on the sand shore, we gather ourselves for one last time, and go to that place that has no invectives nor translucence, and no need to let things fly. I am here, like the eagle. I am here like the bird that has no flight. There is a wishing in the umbrage of it all. There comes a vast vantage, that settles into the darkness like cheese on a marble bench – like the tutelage of someone of note. And then – magic – like we have never known. Yes, and then?

Washing with sticks, we settle on the Dias, and known the sound of earth to be loud. And then whispering to the sky, we discover something we had not known before. What is here, is here – but what is there, can never truly be there - only in the pejorative do we find that in play. Only in this frame of mind does that happen. Much is believed about this in times of trouble, times of difficulty. There is a chance we will find its effects in nature, effects soon discovered.

There is a gaining, with no perception given. There is wistful turning, turning about the grave of it. Do not stay long. Only as things are in their right position, and in their right motion. Things will celebrate as they are. I embrace a right way to be. Much that is turned over, is turned over to purely to see. There is more to life than the dandelion knows. What is all that we say is sure, is the rough of the rinse, and what's more, the sense of companionship.

Gaining in strength, one foot after the next. There is a lopsided trajectory we need not correct. Everything is in its proper place. We adjust a little of our own idiosyncrasies, and then climb into bed and wait for the pan of time to train our hand again. We launch into life then, like a dragon on the sill. Like a dragon-fly nestled in close. Like something we had never seen before, only dreamt of, and soon forgotten. Yes, indeed.

Much in line with what has gone before. Much in line with what we expect. There are places in the soul we shouldn't see, and we have seen them. There are places that shouldn't be told of them, and we have told of them. There is a likeness to the clouds here, and there is a likeness to the sky. And there is a likeness to all that flourishes on this crying globe. We can never really see that clearly – except in one thing; love. But this is just for memories sake.

Why do we cry in the dead of night? Why do we say no, when yes is the answer that is sought? What becomes of the stallion, when the stallion bolts? What do we say of our lives, when each beaten track we travel down is as difficult as the last. Why do we keep positioning ourselves, when to do so is to wed ourselves to fate. When to keep with this when it is to lose more than enough. We will give to remoteness one more time, and then let go of things as they are – one more time

And then, like a rainbow that never subsides, muscle mass that never diminishes. A lost castle that is sterling in victory. A lot that comes to us all – in every way – pure or cheap (or both). We sing a song here, one for the time that has elapsed. It is of you and me and our fawning. Is this what we shouldn't ask? Is this what the dawn does not inquire about? Is this what we thought could never happen, in the weave of it. There is the notion to think of – that will be as much.

Foraging, and yet still. A life-line, and all that will perplex. A tremendous shadow that is only half dark. What we once saw, but could not give the gist of. What we once saw, but have no time to see again. What we once saw, but are now too tired to feel. What we threw away, but now wish to keep. There is much to see here, and much to council, and much to then applaud. There will be more to come, before we are through. More to come.

A picture in an abandoned art gallery that knows more than we can comprehend. Something special about things, but we don't know why. We get a taste for it after a while, and then we let it go. Best not to see things afloat, or through in anyway. There is something of the belligerent here, something we thought would never come to pass. Don't simply wander, there is like a masseuse here, one to settle all nerves. A tempest before, or after?

Milestones etched in fabric. A crusade, for who knows what. There is magic in these hills. Magic, the source of which cannot placate. There is an engine humming, despite our protestations. We lag, but only because we are allowed to. There is an acre of things to do here, much that seems pedestrian. But at the heart of it, there are things we cannot surmise – and that is dismissed with literal attendance. We will not let the world win.

There are vice-regal regalia's that are limited in scope, if not affection. We ask for perfection, and are given some, despite. We have the difference in mind. The difference in estimates, the difference in control, the difference in expectation. Do not live for this, there is a time, for everything, or everyone. There is a time to thrive, a time to rejoice, a time to eat, and a time to simply be. There is more than enough to see.

What have we grown towards, other than all the efforts of the field? Fields of barley, fields of corn. We listen, but for what? We take hold, but of whom? There is a register, but who takes it down? We know of one thing, life is difficult, but so is much. We have nothing to rest upon, so what do we do now? We rest upon white wings, and know our purchase to be thin. There is a coupling that eases, as it restricts. But what of the pain of it – we will fight.

The sea. The heart. The sea and the heart. Do we digress? – No, towards the centre. How do we hear our own heart beat without a stethoscope – simple, we drive down to the sea get out of our car, and listen as intently as we can. And that is the sound of your own heart. Magic – it is here. I can hear now, in my mind, the lapping of the sea on the sea shore – that is it my heart beat. There is more to be said here, and we will say it.

There are gains, gains and red ink. We long for something else, but have nothing left to please. But that is not true. We have much in our lives. All one must do is look, and lo it is found. All one must do is see, see for the first time. And things will remedy themselves in due course. Much to be said here, much to be delighted by. Wrangle the disc, it causes no pain not impropriety. A method arises that has no brand to pursue. Come now, this causes that.

Chapter 10.

Wishing through it all. Hoping for a better result. There is here a mission to uphold. There is here something we can dance with. And then, like a gathering in the middle of nowhere, we come. It is here we fashion all.

A makeshift machine that tells the time, in breaks of gold. A certain relief from the pomposity of it all. We look forward to things that carry only the wind. There is here nothing we have yet seen. That is enough.

Whistling – there is no other way. Whistling, in light and dark. We consider things true, unless it is stated otherwise. There is a camp in amongst it, that gives directions as it wanders. Could this be it?

And then we wander, as the sinew bites, and the legs simply take us. We have more of what is near. What is near and what is far. There is here a response to the day. We must not concur, only in the dream state – the oneiric.

The heart it comes – the sea it does likewise. Do we see either of them? – Perhaps the sea. But that is okay. We must ride the waves of this sea.

We must put our hands on our hearts, and feel the pulse.

There is here something to describe – it is round and soft, and crimson. It is the world as seen by those who sleep. But when we awaken, what then? We then see our lives in common drama. We must only move a muscle.

Lots to live for – lots to fashion a life out of. And here, where the dance is at its most intense, here we live the brightest. And then, a sound to be free with. It is like something out of a bowl.

We champion only one thing, and one thing only. And that is in doing so, we do not forget the name of it. That is important. That is what makes us, or mars us. Somethings remain the same, and somethings change.

Cracking in, for the life of us, we do not know why. But that stays a truth, much invigorated, and much contested. There are wheels a foot, and tangles to set against. We do feel seemingly aghast at it all.

There is no place like this, no place like the furthest from anywhere. We are happy with the respite wherever we are. And that goes for all of us. There can be no complaints – to be sure of the matter.

Much delight – there is something happening at 9pm, are you ready? How to get there, we will simply walk. Is it close to us? Yes it is. We will walk. Excitement, the gathering of pace. This is what we need.

A wonderful adventure is had by all. And then like a case made of sand - we keep our valuables elsewhere. Do not be concerned at the coming and going of it all. There is a tempest without recourse. We will temper it.

Much that is in the ascendency, and much we have not missed. There is a large foregoing, and then, a smaller one. The sequence of things is not out of touch. The waves. The waves.

A sense of condolence weeps through the tears. And here, where the years wander, but do not go astray, there is a capturing that heartens, and yet does not glean further shores. The testament to the fact is here in-amongst it.

A tiredness creeps in despite the weather. And it is here that the time moves as slowly as it possibly can. And now, we say to you, come for the landing, and stay to be resplendent. There was once a district here, we can surmise.

Do we say our piece to relinquish control, or is it the opposite, where we try and assert ourselves again. There is never a tether to be ashamed of. Never a tether to reproach. Please be one to stand when others sit. That will suffice.

Much pleasure has accompanied us, over hill and dale, through wind and rain, through ice and pain. What is the life of it? – We will never know. We are also unable to tell. A toll too late. A sense of being in calmness – and being calm.

Outside of every known contortion, we sense our time is approaching. This seems strange – or not strange, but surprising – to us who have approached the falconer for guidance. There is now a forum for such things.

There are no lessons left to learn – nothing left to shy away from. There is here, like all places, time to dwell, and time to stay – If you are content in that? There is a crumbling from the corner – we must listen. And from here we will.

There was once a time of treading easily – but not now. There was once a time of playful ease – but not now. What do we have now? We have those things, but they are covered – how do we uncover them? – With spirit.

What is the sea, but a heart? – Pumping
necessary fluids around the earth-body. What is
the heart, but reminiscent of the sea? – Pumping,
pumping, pumping. Here is a close comparison,
one we can revel in.

Be with us now, now that we have time to talk. We
will talk of wonders, wonders of the past –
wonders of the present – and what will be – the
future. Docile, no. Adventurous, yes. There is now
a way in.

A sampling of what comes next. It is meticulous in
endeavour. It shows loquacity from time to time,
but not overmuch. There wrangles impropriety, but
only briefly. We carry our sticks – but we let
ourselves play for one more time.

There is truth here, like a bastion. Each tear from
each cry a wandering. Each sound from a muse, a
journey. Tenacity, and strength of mind, allows
what needs to happen. There will come a crashing
– but we will survive.

Nothing short of excellent. Nothing sort of
disastrous. We come for the stasis, but leave for
the ambivalence. Do not be cautioned, willing will
always help. There can be nothing short of it – we
will revel.

A force to it – we have the template. And here, a magnetism that undulates – with skill and aplomb. Do not carry us too far – we will not go. Do not pull the sled too fast, we wish for a pleasant journey. Ha. Of course.

A whisper, and what is firm grows firmer. We will sprout like a vegetable. And then like whistling we harbour no thoughts, and begin to dream of faraway places. What is this? Nothing but the shelter of something we don't understand.

Misanthrope – tangled. The here and now ensconced. We love to be, and without such, there wouldn't be much left. But do we say to this? What do we say when time redeems its stance, and knows things for the first time.

A short but entrenched byway, one that leaves nothing to the imagination. There comes a sound, one that livens the city streets – unto daylight, unto night. There is now a march that descends from a place unseen. We will see what is to be seen.

Lying flat, we slowly get up, and know the destiny of us all. This knowledge, that is gleaned from the rooftops, will shield us from much – but much comes through. So it is, with tinder and in bulk. Do not change the way of.

The times come – the times go – pitter-patter, pitter-patter. A nervous stretch, and simplicity at the touch. Why is there nothing left of us? Why does the noise we make sound so muffled? We will come, and we will go – just for show.

There is a landline in the trees. There is much to see of things. I will follow where you want to go. And where is that? To the top of things. But where is that? In-between the laughter and the merriment. Choose your course. Things will come.

A forward motion, one that leaves us in the region of light, in the region of day. What are these regions? Do they give a cold shoulder, or do they welcome us as the pariah of sight? We may never know.

Reaching for the midst of it, we find our way there – like marbles in twilight. Like sentences along the way. Like an ambush when you least expect it. Like running up that road – like something unheard of.

Hastening to open our door – we find another way in. And it is here where our souls have become longed for, and our hearts to be opened. A type of merriment greets us, and we simply do not need nor want for anything else.

And then, like a rascal that never diminishes, tender hooks set the world ablaze, and know what we need to keep going. There is pain – yes. But there is also respite – and fun. Come now, let us enjoy ourselves.

A much-needed opining fills the void. And here, the moisture of our tears does not render us vapid, nor out of touch. We come once again, despite ourselves – despite our wandering and wander-lust.

There is a cause to all this – the sea, the heart. Those two things never hesitate. Those two things rush at us. Those two things. We never once have seen the score to settle our nerves. Heart and sea.

A coaching the world does, if we did but listen. A worrying we wouldn't do, if only we did listen. There is a chamber, deep inside all of us, that contains all we need. It is here, we catch hold, and never let go.

A tradition, that has us falling into life, one hand at a time. We will always come here – for swimming, and lounging, and relaxing. We cannot be the turnstile here, for there are many people.

There is in each of us a part that holds down exertion, and knows how it trims. Obligingly, fate will show how this is done. And a-one and a-two, and here we go - method and unbecoming shade.

There is a globe of the world that sits at the edge of things. In this globe, and in its rotation, there lies everything we could possibly need. How to find it though? We know this will be hard, but the rewards are endless.

A mystery that never stops. A mechanism that does not tame itself. All the bells and whistles. Contagion in a well, well-springs for life. And now, we come, crescent in hand. Cresent before us – and away.

Much ado – but much less bravado. We seldom see the outskirts of the tenacity of things. That's okay, we cannot alter the rainbow for anyone. A distance that luxuriates in its own sense of being. We are not at a loss.

Attributing what must be liaised with. And now we know for sure, but what is the cost? What of sand between our toes? What of the developments at hand? We will not shirk, for anything or anyone.

There is here hope – but what form does it take? Who has it? What are its benefits? There is here, also a tempest, that lingers only as far as we will let it. How far is that? Only too much to agree.

A wish band or bracelet – does it come with us – in second or third motion – is this what we see, just before we sleep. There can be nothing else, nothing else to it. And then with gusto, one trick more.

There is now a wind that we have not seen nor heard before. And in this wind, there is a heart, there is a sea, and in this way, there is more than we can believe. We must not remind ourselves; we can do what is best.

A mix of messages – staged, but not contrived. We learn from every bit. The signal in the tail tells us that time is not curtailed. Makeshift surroundings let us dispose of the grandeur. We will not frolic.

Come into life, I hear you say. Come into the less that pallid mosaic. There is heart here, there is contiguity, that never knows breath – that never opens sharply, nor strongly. Where is the palace?

Touch, and do not spoil – a random signage comes through, and affixes itself to wondering hearts. The breath we use here is not for reminiscing. But we call for action – action for what? – For it all.

Licence to get underway. And then like shards, we conquer. Like the wrong way, but like endeavouring, the mistaken and the angry pull a mighty punch. Ringing like blows from heaven. We wander down – and then through.

A tight space, one which is tricky to navigate. A tight space, we linger here like the night. We have all the might of all the journeys never unravelled into one. That catches the rain when it comes down.

Fostering companionship. Being tutored by one of the greats – being neither here nor there. Being stronger still. We love what we have become. And that is stronger still – never fall down – never.

Tightrope – and tightrope walker. Messages to be sent, and then copied. A looking forward, but not behind. There is a case for rectilinear motion. And then, something from the maelstrom. We will cover ourselves.

The ocean is locked into motion, just as the heart is. One gravitational, the other biological. There is a new time we cannot wrestle against. But it is here that we relinquish pride, and know ourselves to be worthy.

A lot has come this way, through fire and ice. We do not delve into each other's destiny. But what we do will surprise – and that is open ourselves to the night, and have dreams and hopes pinned on yore.

A capitulation to one another, that sounds as if it was out-striped by the hollowing. Do not bend yourself with more than can be wound. There is a trick to this – and we will play it. Do not bend close to the origin point. There is much to see.

Fawning, and waving. Not knowing the task. Not knowing which way to go. Not knowing that everyone that has commenced has found love. And not knowing that everyone who has commenced sensed more.

Blood and raiments – trickle down. What we thought would be too high, has turned out to be perfect. We like to think that the ground below us is soft, and will cushion our fall – to a certain extent it is – just watch out for the hardness.

A white in the eyes, deflects our blow. We see, but are not perturbed. We long, but do so out of fervour. And then like a stake in the middle, we eat away. Do what you must – that is important. More so, very important.

A wandering that gathers pace. Someone attaches a work of art in a stair well – the work depicts a tropical scene – of the breaking sea. I stand for minutes at a time – and I am calmed.

Catching on the rungs of it, we let ourselves know what is here, and what is there. Do not be disconcerted, the last of it rings out above the maelstrom. There is a certain whimsicality that delivers the no-man's land of desire and feeling.

I believe in the sighs of the all-or-nothing, and the incredible weighing of townships and the be all and end all of fate. What is left of us, I hear you ask. There is a moon that is full tonight, let us be something special.

The treatment space had much of what is needed, but much that wasn't. We limp in, and take a seat. Only for this occasion do we come. Only for what is next do we even have a splattering of effect. This is what it is for.

The daring we have, does not fail to announce itself, is that which the bravado of life will not curtail, if it can avoid. Much space to play the larrikin. Much space to ride the envelope through and through. We will march with much insistence.

Grinding out, of this place and then here. I look onto untimely reaches, untimely plateaus – just simply untimely. What do we say of this adventure – more or less? There is a fate that has the sound ringing in our ears. We will run.

Do we delight in all that has gone before, or do we stand firm, and rig out a mast and a deck and all the rest? This is what we should do. And then we are ready, ready to roam free, on the sea of unknown abandon.

A tailing inward, but not outwards. A flight to some other shore. What is it we seek, other than this, other than that? We know where life will take us, but we are not perturbed. It will cause an aspect of concern, however – but that is okay.

A convergence of things we don't understand. A lapsing that is heartfelt. A tremendous outcry the does not belittle. There is fervour in my voice, it descends to reach, and then is away. We will not pretend.

Chapter 11.

Considering the options, we know where the sea breaks. It is here, and through, and away. Do not be belligerent, the test will soothe. There is hope, hope to see things anew. There is a mass of indices that pour no cloth. There is here and there is now. There is what we have thought, and then nothing of it. A treasure to be seen. A missive that hurdles the climb. I will say to you one more thing. The more is at the meeting point – we must salvage it.

A random type – we feel no breeze, but what of that, we launch into the sounds of life, only to let go, and once again. Things seem viscous here - newly arrived, and affected by the travels of greater hardship. Do what is not adhered to by the promised and brave. We can always be close to our heart, no matter what. I am a firm believer in the constellations, and all that fits the hat of the greater temperament. We will fill the void.

Hanging out the coils that do not last. Being insipid, and then strong. Never calling the way through. Always being, but by never enough. Are you the steeple and the consecrated? Do victims come, and lieges warrant? We will say tremendous things, and not be afraid of what is said? There is a sound here, more like a play, than anything else. And it is here where we do our best work – all we need is a treat, and of we go.

Leaving the door open. Go out for the rainbow of it. Seeing something more. It seems as if the 'we' have a hold of it. It seems as if the impartial inquirer has nowhere to go. What is this we find? What is this we salvage? Is it something new, or old. The muse in the distance is singing for us. What do we do when the earth does not face us? It comes we know, but does it shy away? We will hear more than we can mould. That much is a boon.

We tag along, not knowing where we are going. But that is okay, somethings are meant, and this is one of them. We have a choice along the way – left, or right? We choose to smooth the brambles of a life lived. But what is that to do? We only know when we do it. That is the limitation of us all. Before we are tired, we have something else to say – and what is that? We cannot crouch too tightly, it is not our way. And then, a heart-felt applause.

There is a space, between things – both animate and inanimate – a space where life is never harvested. And here, where we once lived, there is a cascading of all this vigilant. Never seeing the test for what it is. I will embrace you, like never before. And then, like raindrops on a tin roof, we gather for one last time. It is pleasant to be in this company again. But we only know how to come back now. But then – the greatest of arcs.

Marching through, and then coming out from under things. We pay our price, and then the world turns that one more time. We don't distance ourselves anymore, for anything, nor anyone. We laugh at the spattering of fairy lights that decorate the hall. Are we ones to collide in unison, and never roll ourselves back? There is a space back here, where the mannerisms of an age take shape. And when we live, we do so with gusto and aplomb. There is never anything to worry us by.

And now, where we find ourselves, we come around again. There is a lot to life – meaning; that is our lot – or meaning; and a lot, a great many things. Come and see how much more is required. In this height of trees, there is a lesson to be learned. Simple things are held, and complex things are balanced. Is there a fate for all these things – I should hope so. We come again, for what is in need, and what it is that brings hardship. Both are valuable. We will come for them.

Very sharply, we turn again. Very quickly we find our space on the road of things. Where will it end? When will the focus be the homecoming, and not the lyre? When will the mixture of height and silk be so ever remembered. There is now something that can only be reneged by a kindred spirit. Officially there, and through, and what's more abundant. I have seen these things before, on the highway, on the byway. Never enacted, always hinted at.

Swimming in a sea of it. Swimming end over end. We placate ourselves when there is nothing left to do. Hold on to the banister, fate is here. There is no time to be admonished – no time to set sail. We have as we have clasped. We have as we have known, and as we have given solace to. The dream, the dream – do we ponder as most, or do our lashings subside on the backs of unruly men. Do not contain what is not here. We are allowed to wallow, and that we do.

High above, down below – in-between, through and through. There is nestled here something of the ilk, but what we can tell of it, apart from who sulks who. There is time enough to find the whereabouts of all known fashionistas, as they warble together as a flock. Please place undue pressure on the fastings of men and woman of the solace, they have no place here. When we know that we are in alignment, grand things are possible.

A suitably large applause – but for what? For this, the settling of an age-old question. What is this question? We cannot tell you, it is written on silk, on water – ink on water. Can we decipher it? I don't know. But look here, we have the tenor of it. There was once a place, how long ago…? That will have to do. Conquistadores come – there is room. And when we lumber forward, on two feet, we have done more to sally-forth than most.

A wishbone in tidal pools of life. Come now, our host has forgotten himself. Where was I – ah yes, there is a key amongst it that knows only skies, and how to unlock them. And then, like a chamber in release, there is a sound that follows. We linger away, and see ourselves wandering through the veritable and the furrowed of brow. Can we simply move around as usual? There is no telling what would happen. And then, in line, a refurbishment.

Witnessing history, we come full circle. We love what it is we do, and what it is we do we love. Gathering pace, the momentum here is audacious. Catching a rhythm to the end of things is a respite we shouldn't have. Beckoning and wading through, systems are a plenty. And then, like rice on paper, we see ourselves once more. This is where we should tie our horse – or maybe let it wander. A seance where we learn a thing or two. Much to be laughed at, but much not.

I will give glasses to the wicked, so that they may see. There is something about this that we aren't aware of – but we must; and we will, and nothing else to it. We laugh, but what is it about the sanctioning of rights that tells us all we are needed. Give more than your share, and the energy you have will not be wasted. The further we talk, the more eccentric we get. The further we loom, the more unbecoming. We have time for one last thing – let us do it.

There is news from afar. It states that war is dead, long live peace. There can only be these words in amongst it. We tell ourselves in the morning we have tried. But then, what do we do next? Sanctions of need, sanctions of life. And now, without much as a throw of the dice, we canter into something fresh. What do we say, what do we feel? We hope for forgiveness, but what is that, without the need to try – hyperbole wins.

Sanctimonious and away. Short and narrowing. Cautious and believing in the sand. There is here something that tails, off into the distance. Let us remember how far we have come. Let us see what is ahead. Let us not tarry. Let us remain calm as we go. There is a ship in the distance – we will reach for it, and know it to be a friend. It will take us far. Each step of the journey is laced with difficulty. But that is okay, that is what we need. We will be.

Vestiges of time – shreds of space. And here where the fathoming of night-time arrays catch on to give a colour to life, there is a special envoy waiting in the wings. We have neither the wherewithal nor the compulsion to act in accordance with the wind. Never believe so. This much is true. I sense without a tarry as all things, there is desire. But what of life, yes. What of the mire – yes and yes. Mostly we come when we can.

The heart – the sea. Do we hear them? Is this where we find them, over here? Do they sound the same? They both can be reached – should we include the horizon, and the sound it makes at dawn? That's it, what a beautiful thing. And now we set sail, surrounded by the blue, the sounds of the ocean in our cabin – we listen to our partners heart – what a thing to do. The coursing of the wind, the waves – small for now. This is life.

Much to do, much to undo. In the puzzle is the fragment. And here, like servitude we spring. And then, like a spring embrace, we become writ large. It is not ours to determine, nor ours to warrant. I will make things as I wish. There is a dearth of accompaniments – but we will circle. There hosts more than our fair share. We love as we are needed, and that is enough to sense the position of it. When the rain comes, we will know.

We are acclimatised to things, and here we shout our last. We storm by the maelstrom, and have time for nothing else. But what of this, such that it comes in unison and without remorse. We will have it in full. But there is more here to say – and more here to do. We won't listen to the sparks of the memory anymore. It is as if the side-line has taken centre stage. Come forward so the crowd can see you. We want you here.

A solemn procession that tells not the time, nor which way to go. There is something in the wind – we will have our fill finding out what it is. There is a feeling of aghast that litters with milk and honey. Do not gain weight, we are already full – full of life. And then, something wells – is it the future? Is it the past? – We don't know. But we are short of breath, but we come inside, to be sure. Silence reigns, as the door hinge creaks. We will unleash.

There is something in this journey that perplexes. Who is the king of airs and graces? What do we say when we find out? There is now a finite time to discover. Including that which never marches. There is a distance here we hadn't thought of. We hark back to days unknown – and then with a mighty cry we leap. The air feels so fresh here – we will not make amends. But that is all we can say, before abeyance and contrition.

Request a ransom, and see what transpires. Accept the best, and have the where-with-all to run with the tigers. There is here a news amendment, we link arms, and see where it takes us. In the middle, we come. At the edges we come. And then, like firebrands we soar. There is nothing to waste here – only that which comes in threes. There can only be what we need. And then like a solemn mass, we come. To detour like the average. We leverage nothing.

There is a force of nature that has as its core an intensity that does not drift. We must harness this intensity, and in doing so give life to the trees, and all of the world. But this is a course of action that is surely not needed. Maybe in a times gone by. But here and now, we are ready. Mist – the dome which is the sky. Alongside and through. The stars – the horizon, what is best. We come here again and again, and in here lie the tendrils of resurgence. They take no sidestep.

There is an action here worthy of four. And in this motion, comes a solid sound. We have never heard a more insistent whining. There is tape here to hold us together. And when we are done, a forwards motion to help keep us clear. Our head is the same as always, but what of the waist, and legs and the feet? They come to. We send ourselves to all parts of the world, never to be reticent, never to let out a shout. There is here a little of the brisk. We have come.

There is a guard to be as we need. Lovingly erected, like silk in oil and tethers. There is here a group of newcomers, ready to be on deck as we need them. And we need them. The soul of it comes like fashion in the wings. We love the way this goes. There is a bounce now in the steps of a thousand teachers teaching. Do be kind, there is enough to say. This much is now clear. We curtail anything of the rosemary and the thyme. There has been much said – and we have said it.

Wrangled and put in a case. We will need that later. What have we now but supervenience. And then, like a ship that has no sails, there will remain an aghast captain. But what does this say of the pride of things? We know that chances will prevail. There are things risked upon, that give only soil. But that is okay, wandering placates. There is a message to all and sundry – be brave, give effort, and you will soar.

There is enough to see through, and more than that, there is enough to be through. There can only be what is next. There can only be what we know. And despite all of this, we wander, and have our heart set in steel. There is no other motion than this. There can be no other motion. We stick to the semblance of things, and then through, and then over. What is this dust that has settled on ancient mantlepieces? We will dust it off, carefully at first, and then with a more vigorous motion.

What is this up ahead? What do we see? Is it the distance to the all-or-nothing that sits in straights of blue and yellow. We come, but for what? There is always time, always the machinations of what is real. A constancy that evicts, evicts all that have ever trodden on a goad have seen. Do not choose the centre of things, the periphery is all that is needed. We tend not to worry about the outcome of things, when there is a solid base to work with.

Disposing of the myth, we come again to the position of the stars. We don't tend to see many stars in the night sky from a city. But they are there. We simply must go to the rural regions – and there they are – so many to see. And then like a flagship that doesn't know when to stop, we come down, not in the way it has been portrayed – but differently, without mirth, with style, and divergence. Do we hear what will come? We can if our ears are right.

There is never a silence to beckon more than it should. We have speech, but what else do we need? There is a crescent moon in tasteful array. There are machinations that do not seal. We have here only what doesn't fit. And here, like a burgeoning of all out painting – artists come and engage on a project that has never seen the surface of this world of ours. Something grand enough to be potted in soil. But what of the transit? It will near.

There is a chance for us. A chance to do what is here. And we will do it, and do it in this fashion. The majesty of all, that has yet to be conquered, and then hit through, and beyond. Give us a rise, a rise to the hills. We come to land in plaintive song. Do not be the one to rally, that is already here. Come for all that come after us. They will see not as we see, but through new towers, and makeshift abodes. What is their effect? To enliven.

Walking to who knows where – all we know is that we are gaining momentum. And then like fog, we drift, and have as our station all that time will give. Despite the way forward, we are making good time of the journey. We have come prepared, and know that there is density ahead. Never once willing to wander – except now. The path seems so well trodden, we might have to go for an explore. We set of, and realise what we should do. We are there, we have found the path.

Drying moist gum leaves, we now see our way forward. There is a loss of time, and something which resembles a paddock with criss-crossing paths. We linger, but not long enough. We are never this way inclined. But what an adventure, miss-mashing, unheard ties, dense misnomers, and all that the valley will bring. There is now a palpable feeling that the worst of the journey is behind us. We think ourselves lucky for a moment, and then continue on. That is true.

Much to our chagrin, the way forward deepens. But then as quickly it recedes, no part of it resembles what it was. We then again come to an impasse – but what do we do? We borrow what we can to make this journey as comfortable as it can be. And then, like windows in sand – it passes, and what we find is a coolness in the breeze. And what we find gives us time to reflect – reflect where we have been, what we have done, and where we can go from here.

Sensing no danger, not of the current, we move in unison, down through the wisps of vine, down through marching pariahs, and out again. Is there time now to seek congress, congress with all those who travel this path. There is never enough to say I am thirsty. This time at least is the time of wolves. But we caution ourselves, never to seek regress. I will have more of the way of it. What is more, is that sense will reign, in shards and in what must be.

Compulsion – what is that? Gravity, and a sense of awe. We have found what we are looking for. There is here a place to shelter, and here a place to be taught. Do you really feel like you're alive? Is this the remedy to be given. I hope it is. And now like a thoroughfare uncoupled, we move in ways of silk, ways of dandelions. Come for the treasure of it – stay for the vines. We move in gracious tones, never thinking of the crux of it – however we will remember it.

The sea, the heart – what more can be said? We dance a dance in fabricated nuances. And in this we mimic the sea – and our hearts beat even faster. But which is quicker? The heart or the sea? The answer depends on how much the heart is exerted. An exercised heart beats fast – but the sea in a storm goes quick as well. It must be said, I believe, that they are equal. The sea and the heart have equal energies under different circumstances.

There is here a whispering that knows only fate. And in this we love. In this we have faith. In it is here we know ourselves. Don't be too kind, there are limits. And then, like a raging interval, we measure ourselves in time to chosen brass. There lifts a finger, that is then straightened, and relaxed. Much to see, much to know. Much to want to believe in – if that can be said. Capturing the motif, and sliding it through. There is not a thing to waste.

Compassion, it is key. Without it, we are nothing. It comes to us in waves, and is thus resplendent as it arches, until our backs run with sweat. Do we find that little bit extra in our movements – what is this? There is time for all of this. Time to reach the limit, time to fashion a tree branch. Time to believe in unbelievable things. and then like the well wishes of a stranger, we pass, and are passed. Do you really want to see what life is like? Of course we do – then come.

There is time for much – but when time runs out – look out. There is now enough time to keep things going for the foreseeable future. But one day time will simply be tamed, that much will happen. But what of the well-spring and the vision, they will win. We laugh, but there is no time for laughter – this is serious work, humid and in line with what is known. We catch ourselves, only so we do not break. We will enjoy ourselves to lessen what we can only do.

Melee with ghosts. A chapter out of the book we are reading. There is harmony in the wings. There is something special to the portents we wrap up against. Never once have we seen this. There is a turn of speed we just can't seem to grasp. And then, like an expanse of air, we come down swiftly, and know our journey to be true. Do not be concerned, much is written, that aims for life. Do not wish for the clouds until they are here. We can sense it.

A lesser-known fact – the clouds give us much pleasure as the dawn. And it is here where we find our release. This is what we live for, and find in the sides of eddies of air. There is something special about this, that readies itself for the conch-shell, and what comes next. Some, like us, have the mist here. There comes a marching to this effect, but not a drowning out. There is life in these parts - parts of these climbs. We can only soar, that is the rule of it.

There is never anything to fear. Because here, much rests on what is ready. And much sees itself already gone. We barely have time to look, and, shock, it is here. I reach up, and climb that way we have always climbed. There is a way to do things, and we have found it. There is rice in the waiting, would you believe. And then like gargoyles that stave off all, much to be missed about. Convex, and then concave – there is always a mystery to be beheld.

A rise in the number of folds and creases in the table cloth. We count them to, and see which half has the largest number. Not just to pass the time, but to keep things going. Do we sort ourselves to into much needed categories. Things that never go to waste. We will find ourselves again here. This much we hum to, and this much we see. I cannot gain more of the approach than we have ceded today. There is a language all of its own – we will see what it says.

There is coldness here, like the streets have never known. But what we partake of is not that, but all the wind can carry on her voice, and through her wings. We have ennobled her and given her strength – this much is sure. What of the rest of the earth – a keepsake, and cushioning. We will lock together, and see what happens. There is a majesty to this that we keep finely tuned. What more can we say? What more can we do. Vipers see the edge of things.

Chapter 12.

The sea – on this day, was rough. But in our hearts, there was calm. This is sometimes how things go. But we have never seen the sea like this. When we hear, all we hear is the sea – we cannot hear our hearts.

A vestige of what we once where. And we use these thoughts to throw our fears out of the stratosphere. And then like a matchstick unused we stumble forward. There is only what we have to keep us going.

A motion that never truly sees. There is rest here, and the time it takes. Come though the way of it – we must settle in. Settle in to something special. Come now, do not be terse, we linger, and know our direction will last.

A belonging that leads the way. What is left, when troubadours have their say? There is something else to consider. Something that no force of nature can witness. And here where the noise of life is high – we match it with our hearts.

A lot that is not lost. A feeling that does not dampen. A mixture of sense and nonsense. What is left, we cannot say. What remains, we all stand to attention. There is a wrangling in the mist. We come for more, and indeed, less.

A lassitude that never minds. A work we do. We call beyond ourselves, and know that in this action, there is contained the whole of something very peculiar. What is needed, is a cart to drag it all away. This much will do.

Sometimes something is brought, that rounds out the life of the person to whom it is brought for. And then like a realm of science, things just make sense. We will never truly know why – but that is okay – just as well.

And here, where the sand never mentions its name, there is a guardian that believes in things just as we do. But here, our hearts do not beat, in time to the fashion. What is more, we see ourselves in mists of grey, mists of white. We will settle.

A festivity in the ranks. There is life here, something we haven't understood until now. There is life amongst the ruins – amongst the ruins of it all. We cannot withstand the fumes until we have gone.

I see myself in shades of blue, shades of ochre. And then, a certain condolence that only hides its face when it can. Do not be dismissive, the tables have turned towards us, and then through, up and away.

I have never thought of this – in the darkest forest – in unpeeled light. I see myself dragged to consciousness. And it is here that I let go, and have the sense to carry on. We must not linger – it is too tempting.

There is a belief, that the world is older than we know. And in this belief, comes the temptation to count out the years it has been here. But we should not – nay we must not. It would be cruelty to do such a thing – we will make it.

A forwards motion. This is what we have. This is what we marshal. And in that stirs a fountain, whose water is like ice, and whose needs are a condition of the rest. We call on our brethren to open their doors, and let us in.

There is a time, but never a place, for all that goes along – along the road to neverness. We sing, we cry, we undulate, we have figures, at dusk, and then at sight of first light, a new tendency awaits. We are there, to say the least.

How could we ever sing about this? How could this be a part of our vocabulary? The sea is here –

our hearts are beating, what is left will have us bleating. And like a tangent, we step to it.

Crucial and in step, all is in readiness. Come now do not flinch, the signs only will for us. Do we come now, come now for all. We consider ourselves in luck, in grand luck. This much we can say. This much we can do.

A feature of the wind is to cool. And in this, there is life. Life beside the wanting of it. And then, like a solace that has only the power of hearts. We know what we must do. We must unravel the farce for what it is.

Aghast, and awash – awash and aghast. We move forward slowly, and with all that is with us, and all that can be gleaned. Do not gather speed with us – there is no withholding, a thimble full of blood beckons to us. There now.

Masterful, and with taste, the gleam of the loom moves straight ahead. There is nothing left to say, almost nothing left to do. Can we reach for it – in the ounces that are left. We hear ourselves cry, and it is done.

A mission in trails, we have got what we need, and now proceed. There are maps here, and cauldrons to be had. We will have what is said,

and say what is had. An epiphany marks the spot.
We will now rise.

A vestige of the horizon. Systematic change.
Ablutions that never bight. We came here
despondent, but have left resolved. And when we
come again – this resolve will help. This much I
can say.

There is something in the deepest night –
something that cannot be seen or heard. But it is
here, where the magic of a life lived to the brim,
here we must stake our claim. But what is that do,
where sense and repeated nonsense intertwine.

We have fashioned an entire world. One made up
completely of two things – a sea, and hearts. And
here there is no distinguishing which is which –
they both pulse, they both undulate, they both
move with appropriate sound. Great.

And then, like fire and ice, we see ourselves
launching into the briskness of it all. And without
fear of injury of any kind we hear our former
selves give way, and we long for the embrace we
never had.

A scene above, and a scene below. Do we catch
what we need to keep going – catch it from the
sky – or do we luxuriate in untold forms – untold

ways. We never seemed so far away. This will
cool our thighs, cool our hearts.

Much to amaze. Much to move with. Much to
contend with. Much, and mostly intertwined with.
And then, like a feeling we never had, there
comes a sadness – one we are attuned to from
the very beginning. Do not blush. We come.

A lot like we first thought – only stronger – only
within the normal bounds of ringing to. I have
heard more than I can see. And with that much
remains abandoned. Do not recognise the sea,
and what you have heard with adjust against you.

High spirits, low hearts – this is not the way to be.
Viscous and absolved – clenching down on the
wind. We arch for the future, and have our souls
for the past. Do not congeal the play, it is not
ready. We always must dive.

A flabbergast reality, but one that gives. We have
no condolences but what is left? Is this all we do –
follow the lead? Fortitude, and a world away. This
much is clear. We must not belittle the stars.
Come now, we should not force.

What have we said of ourselves that's not out of
kindness. This must bring festivities to the round.
Are we the ones to let the forest free? Does the

thumping sound from the centre of the earth mean its weight? To this very marsh we do bend.

What is stronger than this? What brings its nerve with it? What is like the semaphore, only less involved? We gather now in shifts of shadows, in the near and far – we will pursue nothing else.

Matching weight for weight, we lug ourselves through the estuaries of yore. And what we find there will amaze. Here we come to listen. Here we come to fold on down the line. Mesmerising will excite.

There is much to be seen here. But do not remember too much. For in the laugh, are all the soul can bear. Newly found lynchpins, that do not harvest a grain. We are here, where we want to be. There is no thought to move.

Forever treading, forever bristling. What we find has only half a sheen. We are ones to envisage – and bring with us the night-time embrace. And here despite the merriment, we sit and wish the world a merry journey.

What must we see, if we are to really see? What must we do, if we are to really do? There is doing, and seeing, but something more also. There is the

link to life, that must never stop. We are
weathered but not beaten.

Alternating high fashion, and low. In this
movement the waves have as their dreaming all
the wisps of sorrow that have ever been. But what
of the mast-head, what of the tether? There is in
this a mysterious announcement that only
accompanies the light, and yes, now the fight.

Do we say here – all or nothing? All that can
change, all that can be again and again. There is
something in this, that lingers in the gloom –
words on silk, words on the wire. We will persist
right now.

We will never stop, not until it rains on the shards
upon which we write. And then, like umbrage in
the middle, umbrage on the side, umbrage down
below, an umbrage above - we will mix it with the
best.

Coursing through like never before – I will allow it
– coursing through like never before – we scream
out, out of heart, out of sea – out of all that will be.
We are here to combine heart and sea – and all
that shall not waver

Feeling on top, the waves that carry us do not
falter. The waves that carry us, come above in

rapidity. There is a tension here, that likes no fire – the feels no embers. That comes back again, in crescendo.

Likely, and unlikely – provoking the same. We miss as we do no arrows. And here where the missive tells no tales, the impact is great. We fall aside, and wake as if it was dawn. Come now, awake.

Heralding more than we hoped. A witness to the breeze. Giving what it takes. A feeling of reverence. There is more at stake than we could possibly imagine. We will depart, but how soon? This much we will know. In good time.

Vectors and anchors, a nightly reminiscence. We will take leave of things, before it is too late. But what of the sand? Does it come to announce? But what? How do we send it off? How does it come to be? There will be a flurry of activity.

Engrossed in the weave of it. Engrossed in way of it. There is something we do not understand. There is something we can only capture in parts. Something that lauds as it builds. Something we have yet to silence.

When we see ourselves in depths of the dark, where we no longer have to cherish. It is because here there is no visage to celebrate – no tide to tame – no sense to imagine. We are like life personified but not envisioned.

What have we seen, but what is. What have we felt, but what will come. And then, without a single mis-understanding, we snatch at fate – and see her ride the waves of the nuanced king. And in this, we find our way.

And as if the floor was no longer painted, we gather what it is that holds us close, and then we know of the life that could be ours. And then like a rattle in the sweep of it, we come to gather the steel we need to put inside us.

Nightly, and without rhythm, we are perplexed at the lack of attention. But what do we say, when the dysphoria doesn't budge? All we can do is pray to the dawn – a thing that in fact holds much weight.

Turning around, oh so slowly. And here where the mannerism is in tune, much goes to the centre. I will open many locks for you. Many gateways to the beyond. And here, where the moisture in the air is not of our making, we breathe again.

There can only be one way forward, and that is to see the rose on a lady's back, and have it rise ever so slightly – and then simply follow it, from now till then. And when we open our eyes, nothing left – except all.

Mystery in the bubble. A kind of knot that never returns. I will love what it is that keeps us going. It is something ethereal – something I cannot understand. But that is fine, we dream of light, and have it come cascading through and over.

We have been remiss in the levelling of stone bridges. It is here we fight for our lives, and know that each of our inner selves rejoices in the difficulty of it all. We have more to say, and more to be willing by. Here, and above.

When the wind blows, it does so from the west. When the sand comes in, it does so from the sea (south and west) There is a lot to do, and a lot not to do. Where is our heart? Is it by the sea, watching and waiting?

An absence that doesn't fold. A need that doesn't unfold. There is life in these tenures, life that never misses, life that seeks a quarter – but none is given. We are merry-sent. And then, aspiring towards – and then?

A lasting appraisal. I have more than a sense of it. Go now, to the line in the sand, and have it dawn in branches. There is a laughter where there was once a tangible sense of it. We have come for the relief – we hope to find it here.

Listening intently to what the clouds have to say. And it is here where we are unsure. We could go back, or we could go forward – or we could have stasis, all to ourselves. This could open the window for us.

Sorting through the debris, of a life lived in passion. What we come to believe, is nothing out of the ordinary. But what that is, has the potential to lift us beyond and outside the boundaries that never were there anyway.

A segment of a larger whole. Something closer than we might expect. There is here now, a line in existence, something that we do not know of. And here, where the trudging we do breaks to the mould, much of the same, and all that will be.

I have hope for something to carry me away, on pinions of learned desire. But that which has come, does not renege. And you can't argue with that. There are places in due course that we would love to visit – I will leave them to your imagination to see.

A wry smile – one that we can't imagine of ourselves. We begin our journey, through dry grass and leaves, through the parkland, over dale, over hills, across streams – and away. There is here something special. We will see it.

An effort, to be where we should. And it is this effort, that makes us or break us. Despite the languid turn, and despite the curtailing of summer suns, we catch ourselves in readiness. Do not linger – and off we go.

Fashion yourselves a mosaic, and come for the ride of rides. Do not be the one to transport yourself through linings of grey, lining of white. Come that extra turn of speed will be handy in what comes. Do not relish, simply away.

Searching, but searching for what? Searching for all that touches the sky, and all that falls through. We have no sense of what we are worth, all of us. So let us now combine our search with a walk, and mention to ourselves, yes, we have come.

There is now a chance riding on the wind. We course through, and send ourselves flying. Do not enter here, there is a high degree of activity. This is the way to proceed with us. It seems as if the soul had gone missing…

Halo, and the landscape beyond. Have the last thought you have, that of good times, and times that have depth. To combine the two, is better. And then in constant rotation from the sun, we navigate our way to elsewhere.

The embrace of time. What is it enough of? What can we see of it, when it is here? There is a steep incline here – what should we do with it? What should we say of it? How long will we be? A cushioning, and the science of it.

Walking step by step. Is this the way to go? It can be one way, but can't we also find our balance after ten steps? And then we can walk down to the sea, and bring our stethoscope – and hear the heart – hear the sea.